Tips and Tricks
in
INTERVENTIONAL CARDIOLOGY

Second Edition

Shuvanan Ray
MD DM FSCI FSCAI FACC
Chief of Cardiac Intervention
Fortis Hospitals
Kolkata, West Bengal, India

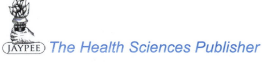

JAYPEE *The Health Sciences Publisher*

New Delhi | London | Panama

Jaypee Brothers Medical Publishers (P) Ltd.

Headquarters
Jaypee Brothers Medical Publishers (P) Ltd.
4838/24, Ansari Road, Daryaganj
New Delhi 110 002, India
Phone: +91-11-43574357
Fax: +91-11-43574314
E-mail: jaypee@jaypeebrothers.com

Overseas Offices
J.P. Medical Ltd.
83, Victoria Street, London
SW1H 0HW (UK)
Phone: +44 20 3170 8910
Fax: +44(0) 20 3008 6180
E-mail: info@jpmedpub.com

Jaypee Highlights Medical Publishers Inc.
City of Knowledge, Building 235, 2nd Floor
Clayton, Panama City, Panama
Phone: +1 507-301-0496
Fax: +1 507-301-0499
E-mail: cservice@jphmedical.com

Jaypee Brothers Medical Publishers (P) Ltd.
17/1-B, Babar Road, Block-B, Shaymali
Mohammadpur, Dhaka-1207
Bangladesh
Mobile: +08801912003485
E-mail: jaypeedhaka@gmail.com

Jaypee Brothers Medical Publishers (P) Ltd.
Bhotahity, Kathmandu, Nepal
Phone: +977-9741283608
E-mail: kathmandu@jaypeebrothers.com

Website: www.jaypeebrothers.com
Website: www.jaypeedigital.com

Tips and Tricks in Interventional Cardiology

First Edition: **2015**

Second Edition: **2017**

ISBN: 978-93-5270-087-5

Printed at Sanat Printers

Dedicated to

*My beloved wife
and
my sons Saunak and Sayak
who are a constant source of inspiration*

Contributors

Prithwiraj Bhattacharjee MD DM (Cardiology)
Consultant
Fortis Hospitals
Kolkata, West Bengal, India

Priyam Mukherjee MD DM (Cardiology)
Consultant
Fortis Hospitals
Kolkata, West Bengal, India

Sabyasachi Mitra MBBS
Registrar
Fortis Hospitals
Kolkata, West Bengal, India

Sanjeev S Mukherjee MD DM (Cardiology)
Consultant
Fortis Hospitals
Kolkata, West Bengal, India

Shuvanan Ray MD DM FSCI FSCAI
Chief of Cardiac Intervention
Fortis Hospitals
Kolkata, West Bengal, India

Siddhartha Bandyopadhyay MD DM (Cardiology)
Consultant
Fortis Hospitals
Kolkata, West Bengal, India

Soumitra Kumar MD DM (Cardiology) FCSI FACC FESC FSCAI FICC FICP
Consultant
Fortis Hospitals
Kolkata, West Bengal, India

Preface to the Second Edition

In no time after the release of the first book, I felt that my book was getting old. So much of information is generated and pumped into the interventional world everyday that to include only the most significant bits would demand another edition with much-increased volume. I never thought of making it obese and sloth; rather, after cutting the unnecessary flab, it looked slim and agile; and thus, the second edition of *Tips and Tricks of Interventional Cardiology* is born.

In this edition, we have added two new chapters, both are illustrative as well as thorough in explaining the basics and scientific advances. These two chapters are vascular anatomy and radiological views and the mechanical circulatory support for complex PCI.

We have also thoroughly updated the older views and techniques as for example adding the ultrasonographic use for different access, which may be helpful not only for percutaneous coronary intervention but also for peripheral intervention.

The stents chapter was thoroughly re-written and for difficult subsets, we have introduced treatment of in-stent restenosis (ISR) and use of drug-coated balloons.

Shuvanan Ray

Preface to the First Edition

Interventional cardiology has become an established specialty since its dramatic beginning in 1977, when Dr Andreas Grüntzig read his remarkable paper to the American College of Cardiology Meeting held in Miami, Florida, USA. In India, it came a decade later and spread exponentially through the angioplasty training courses, workshops and meetings held by the pioneers in the field. As a beginner, a young cardiologist having a postgraduate degree in cardiology, which demands extensive information and reading of congenital, valvular and cardiac muscle diseases and trained mainly in noninvasive procedures, looks at intervention with awe and hesitation, and finds it a difficult and challenging subject.

There are extensive textbooks on interventional cardiology at our disposal, which require almost a lifetime to complete; so cannot be advised to cover up all, before one starts intervention. Learning from them should continue throughout the life. Till then, this small handbook, which deals with essential knowledge for day-to-day procedures can help those who want to start intervention as a fellow or an independent operator, as well as the people in Cathlab, such as technicians and nurses, who ultimately form the team, which delivers necessary care and makes the procedure successful.

I thank my Cathlab colleagues, who contributed their valuable observations and knowledge, which helped me to write this book.

Shuvanan Ray

Acknowledgments

Within two years of release, the second edition of the book turned out to be a reality. This became possible due to constant encouragement and enthusiasm of our Cathlab team, especially, Mr Dipankar Sadhukhan (Chief Technician), Sujoy Bhattacharya and Niladri Ghara. They are instrumental in success of many of our projects and protocols. I also acknowledge Mrs Susweta Banerjee (Chief of CathLab Nursing) and her team, our two coordinators Orpita Nath and Lipika Mondal for their support. I humbly acknowledge Dr Yashesh Paliwal (Chief, Critical Care Unit) and Mrs Banani Bhattacharya and Chandrani Chakraborty (Sister-in-Charge, Intensive Critical Care Unit) for their constant help in patient care, without whom the clinical outcome would not have been great. I acknowledge the silent work of Mr Snehasis Biswas for preparation of the manuscript. I am grateful to Dr Sabyasachi Mitra, who single handedly managed to prepare the manuscript, arranged all the figures, tables, flow charts, gave it a proper shape. I wish him all success in life.

Contents

Who Needs PCI
(Percutaneous Coronary Intervention: For Whom?)

■ Soumitra Kumar

Introduction

The objective of percutaneous coronary intervention (PCI) is to deliver maximum clinical gain at the lowest possible levels of risk. The process involves the interaction of a number of factors:

- The training and experience of the interventionist
- Access to equipment and facilities
- The availability of surgical or other supports
- Characteristics of the patient
- Nature of clinical presentation
- Details of the epicardial coronary anatomy

Unusual or high-risk cases may necessitate the collaboration of other interventionists, clinical cardiologists, internists, surgical and anesthetic colleagues in an institutional 'HEART TEAM'. Above all, process of informed consent can be refined if patients can be appraised of a case specific assessment of likely gains and potential risks. The enthusiasm for PCI must be tempered with realization of the following facts:

Potential for clinical gain is real but selective: In stable angina, there is no evidence to suggest that PCI confers prognostic advantage in low-risk patients, and confers symptomatic benefit which can be modest and can attenuate over medium-term follow-up. In non-ST elevation acute coronary syndrome (NSTE-ACS), invasive strategy will benefit a significant, but selected subset of patients only, i.e. those at high risk; and to a lesser extent, those at an intermediate risk only. In acute ST-elevation myocardial infarction (STEMI), prompt access to PCI facilities and appropriately trained staff may be required within a specific time frame in the natural history, if benefits are to be realized.

Performance of PCI often involves some level of morbidity and mortality: All trials comparing PCI with medical therapy have shown a small albeit higher rate of major adverse cardiac events (MACE) in the intervention group, mostly related to complications at the time of revascularization and these have important complications for the patient's perception of outcome and for the consumption of health-care resources.

Recognition of the fact that alternative options exist and may be equally or more effective: Several independent lines of evidence indicate that revascularization will improve prognosis only in high-risk patients with stable angina. Although there are no randomized data providing this, it is known from large registries that only patients with documented ischemia involving >10% of the LV myocardium have a lower CV, and all cause mortality, when revascularization is performed. In contrast,

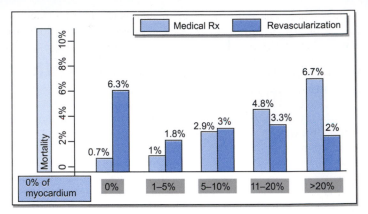

Fig. 1.1: ESC guidelines 2014 (Rx = treatment)

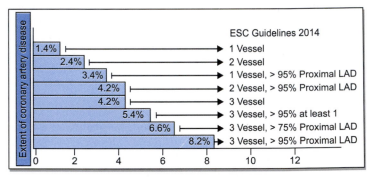

Fig. 1.2: Annual mortality with medical therapy

revascularization can increase mortality in patients with ischemia involving <10% of the myocardium (Fig. 1.1).

Another line of evidence comes from a large prospective angiographic registry that patients with left main stenosis, proximal left anterior descending (LAD) and proximal triple vessel disease, who are known to benefit in terms of prognosis from revascularization had annual death >3% on medical treatment (Fig. 1.2).

Based on FAME-2 Trial, FFR is considered gold standard for invasive assessment of physiological stenosis significance and an indispensable tool for decision making in coronary revascularization. Use of FFR in true catheterization laboratories accurately identifies which lesions should be revascularized, and improves the outcome in most elective clinical and angiographic conditions, as compared with situations where revascularization decisions are simply made on the basis of angiographic appearance of the lesions.

Over the two decades, prior to publication of the five-year outcome of the SYNTAX and FREEDOM trials, approximately 20 trials of percutaneous coronary intervention (PCI) versus coronary artery bypass grafting (CABG) had been conducted. During that period, PCI evolved from plain old balloon angioplasty (POBA), to the use of bare-metal stents (BMS) and then to drug-eluting stents (DES). Similarly, overall results of surgery have also improved substantially, with better medical therapy allied to improvements in anesthesia and surgical techniques, such as increasing use of arterial grafts and off-pump surgery. The most definitive analysis of CABG versus PCI to date (Hlatky et al. 2007), has been a collaborative analysis of individual patient data from ten randomized trials involving 7812 patients. The overall hazard ratio for death with CABG versus PCI was 0.9 (p = 0.12) implying that CABG has no survival benefit over PCI. However, there was a significant reduction in mortality with CABG in patients over 65 years of age (HR = 0.82, p = 0.02) and in patients with diabetes (HR = 0.7, p = 0.014).

Despite the availability of internationally recognized guidelines and recommendations for PCI and CABG in differing anatomical patterns of CAD, it is increasingly recognized that individual practitioners still follow personal preferences even when these are not evidence-based and may be overtly "biased" at times. This is particularly so in the scenario of 'ad-hoc' PCI, i.e. when stenting is performed immediately after diagnostic angiography, and in effect, denying the patient any opportunity to discuss possible surgical options with a cardiac surgeon. This raises questions about the whole consent process and emphasize the need for recommendations for interventions to be overseen by a multidisciplinary "HEART TEAM", rather than an individual practitioner.

Case Selection: A Practical Approach

A structural approach to case selection or risk stratification might consider three elements:

1. *Factors related to nature of clinical presentation:*
   - Acute coronary syndrome (STEMI, NSTE-ACS, cardiogenic shock)
   - Stable ischemic heart disease.
2. *Factors related to clinical characteristics of the patient:*
   - *General cardiac status:* For example, heart failure, hypotension, cardiogenic shock, arrhythmias. Need for elective ventilation or circulatory support (e.g. intra-aortic balloon pump) is a marker of adverse outcome. Postprocedural hypotension or severe bradycardia/tachycardia can precipitate subacute vessel closure.
   - *Peripheral and great vessels:* Atherosclerotic or other diseases of peripheral vessels, e.g. occlusions, tortuosity, unfolding can deny access for catheter of choice or for additional equipment. Risk of catheter-related emboli release to head or neck or peripheral vessel is real. Complications at the vascular access site can result in embolization, occlusion or bleeding. Co-existing hypertension, obesity or systemic anticoagulants can confound these problems.
   - *Renal function:* Chronic renal failure (CRF) is an established risk factor for coronary artery disease and on the other hand, results of PCI at any individual lesion may be less favorable in patients with established CRF. Another important concern for patients with any degree of renal impairment, is that the nephrotoxicity of radiographic contrast can precipitate acute renal failure. Even with precautionary measure such as fluid administration or elective filtration, the scope and duration of any PCI procedure will be limited by the need to minimize exposure to contrast agents.

- *Diabetes mellitus:* The condition is often a marker of more widespread and diffuse coronary artery disease. This pattern of disease is more difficult to manage with PCI, and CABG may provide a better revascularization strategy. This has been evidenced time and again in trials like BARI, ARTS and most recently in Future Revascularization Evaluation in Patients with Diabetes Mellitus: Optimal Management of Multivessel Disease (FREEDOM) trial. The reasons, however, are not fully established, and may extend beyond the simple presence of more extensive disease.

3. *Details of coronary anatomy and characteristics of proposed target lesion(s):* Severity of spread of coronary artery disease, i.e. single versus double versus triple vessel disease should be the first consideration. Next, location of lesions should be considered; not only because of the territory in jeopardy, but also because plaque or other pathologies in left main stem or right ostium or proximal portions of principal vessels increase the risk of vessel dissection or abrupt closure. Due consideration should also be given to lesion characteristics, e.g. branches, bifurcations, calcification and tortuosity. In certain clinical situations (e.g. thrombus laden lesions, saphenous vein graft disease or rotational atherectomy), sequelae of embolization of material to distal vascular bed should be considered. Flow-limiting lesions or occlusive disease in nontarget vessels increase procedural risk. Procedures to a 'last remaining conduit' represent one extreme in this continuum.

Appropriateness of Coronary Intervention

Currently, two major international guidelines namely European Society of Cardiology (ESC) and European Association for Cardiothoracic Surgery (EACTS) in 2010 and the other by ACCF/SCAI/STS/AATS/AHA/ASNC/HFSA/SCCT in 2011, updated in 2012, are available. The latter will be discussed mainly in this chapter to facilitate understanding and grasp of the subject since it summarizes indications under three simple headings namely, appropriate (A), inappropriate (I) and uncertain (U).

Key variables in appropriateness criteria

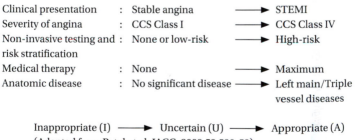

Clinical presentation	:	Stable angina	⟶	STEMI
Severity of angina	:	CCS Class I	⟶	CCS Class IV
Non-invasive testing and risk stratification	:	None or low-risk	⟶	High-risk
Medical therapy	:	None	⟶	Maximum
Anatomic disease	:	No significant disease	⟶	Left main/Triple vessel diseases

Inappropriate (I) ⟶ Uncertain (U) ⟶ Appropriate (A)
(Adapted from Patel et al. JACC. 2009;53:530-53)

Appropriate Indications for PCI in Chronic Coronary Artery Disease (Table 1.1)

- CCS Class I–IV angina with one or two vessel coronary artery disease (CAD) without involvement of proximal left anterior descending

Table 1.1: Appropriate indications for PCI in chronic coronary artery disease

High-risk findings on noninvasive study

Symptoms / Med Rx	CCS class III or IV angina		CCS class I or II angina	
Class III or IV / Max Rx	A	A	A	A
Class I or II / Max Rx	A	A	A	A
Asymptomatic / Max Rx	U	A	A	A
Class III or IV / No/min Rx	A	A	A	A
Class I or II / No/min Rx	U	A	A	A
Asymptomatic / No/min Rx	U	A	A	A

Stress Test / Med Rx	CCS class III or IV angina		CCS class I or II angina	
High-risk / Max Rx	A	A	A	A
High-risk / No/min Rx	A	A	A	A
Int. risk / Max Rx	A	A	A	A
Int. risk / No/min Rx	U	U	A	A
Low-risk / Max Rx	U	A	A	A
Low-risk / No/min Rx	I	U	A	A

Intermediate-risk findings on noninvasive study

Symptoms / Med. Rx	CCS class III or IV angina		CCS class I or II angina	
Class III or IV / Max Rx	A	A	A	A
Class I or II / Max Rx	U	A	A	A

Contd...

Contd...

Symptoms / Med Rx	Stress Test / Med Rx	Intermediate-risk findings on noninvasive study				CCS class I or II angina		Asymptomatic	
Intermediate-risk findings on noninvasive study									
Asymptomatic, Max Rx	Int. risk Max Rx	U	U	U	A	U	A	A	A
Class III or IV, No/min Rx	Int. risk No/min Rx	U	A	A	A	U	U	A	A
Class I or II, No/min Rx	Low-risk Max Rx	U	U	A	A	U	A	A	A
Asymptomatic, No/min Rx	Low-risk No/min Rx	I	U	U	A	I	U	U	U
Low-risk findings on noninvasive study									
Symptoms Med Rx	**Stress Test Med Rx**								
Class III or IV, Max Rx	High-risk Max Rx	U	A	A	A	U	A	A	A
Class I or II, Max Rx	High-risk No/min Rx	U	U	A	A	U	A	A	A
Asymptomatic, Max Rx	Int. risk Max Rx	I	I	U	U	U	U	U	A
Class III or IV, No/min Rx	Int. risk No/min Rx	U	A	A	A	I	U	U	A
Class I or II, No/min Rx	Low-risk Max Rx	I	U	U	U	I	U	U	U
Asymptomatic, No/min Rx	Low-risk No/min Rx	I	U	U	U	I	U	U	U
Coronary anatomy	**Coronary anatomy**	CTO of 1 vz.; no other disease	1 vz. disease of Prox. LAD	2 vz. disease with Prox LAD	3 vz. disease; no left main	CTO of 1 vz.; no other disease	1–2 vz. disease; no Prox. LAD	1 vz. disease of Prox. LAD with Prox. LAD	2 vz. disease with Prox LAD / 3 vz. disease; no left main

Abbreviations: Max, maximum; min, minimum; CTO, chronic total occlusion; prox, proximal; LAD, left anterior descending; Rx, treatment

Source: ACCF/SCAI/STS/AATS/AHA/ASNC/HFSA/SCCT 2012 Appropriate Use Criteria for Coronary Revascularization Focused Update, http://content.onlinejacc.org/article.aspx?articleid=1201161

(LAD) and intermediate risk findings on noninvasive testing. Patient should be on a course of maximal anti-ischemic medical therapy.

- CCS Class I–IV angina with one or two vessel CAD without involvement of proximal LAD and high-risk findings on noninvasive testing. Patient receiving no or minimal anti-ischemic medical therapy.
- Asymptomatic or CCS Class I–IV angina with one or two vessel CAD without involvement of proximal LAD and high-risk findings on non-invasive testing. Patient receiving a course of maximal anti-ischemic medical therapy.
- Chronic total occlusion of one vessel only, with CCS Class III or IV angina on maximal medical therapy and intermediate risk findings on noninvasive study or CCS Class I or II angina with maximal medical therapy and high-risk findings on stress testing.
- One vessel disease involving proximal LAD with CCS Class I–II angina on maximal medical therapy or Class III–IV angina with no or minimal medical therapy and patient having intermediate risk findings on noninvasive testing.
- One vessel disease involving proximal LAD with CCS Class I–II angina on maximal medical therapy and high-risk findings on stress testing.
- Two vessel disease including proximal LAD with CCS Class I–IV angina irrespective of intensity of medical therapy and intermediate risk findings on noninvasive study.
- Two vessel disease including proximal LAD with CCS Class I–II angina irrespective of intensity of medical therapy along with high or intermediate risk findings on noninvasive study, or if on maximal medical therapy, then with low-risk findings on stress testing.
- Three vessel disease (without left main disease) with high or intermediate risk findings on noninvasive study either with symptoms (CCS Class I–IV angina) or asymptomatic, irrespective of intensity of medical therapy. Patients with low-risk findings on stress testing, can be considered appropriate if on maximal medical therapy.

Methods of Revascularization of Advanced CAD

	CABG	PCI
1. Two vessel CAD with proximal LAD	A	A
2. Three vessel CAD with low CAD burden (i.e. three focal stenosis, low SYNTAX score)	A	A
3. Three vessel CAD with intermediate to high CAD burden (i.e. multiple diffuse lesions, presence of CTO or high SYNTAX score)	A	U
4. Isolated left main stenosis	A	U
5. Left main stenosis and additional CAD with low CAD burden (i.e. 1–2 vessel additional involvement, low SYNTAX score)	A	U
6. Left main stenosis and additional CAD with intermediate to high CAD burden (i.e. three vessel involvement, presence of CTO or high SYNTAX score)	A	I

Inappropriate (I)   Uncertain (U)   Appropriate (A)

Proposed scoring system to select patients with chronic coronary artery disease for PCI

Angina Class		Pattern of CAD	
None	0	LMCA	+++++
CCS Class I or II	+	TVD	+++
CCS Class III or IV	++	DVD	++
Post-MI	+++	SVD	++
Symptoms despite maximum medical therapy	+ (additional)	Proximal LAD	+ (additional)

Exercise Test		Comorbidity	
Negative	–	Mild	0
Mild +ve	0	Moderate	–
Strong +ve	++	Severe	–
Post-MI +ve	++ (additional)	Ischemic VT/VF	++

[+] = Positive score
[-] = Negative score
≥ ++++ = Essential indication
+++ = Appropriate indication
≤ ++ = Inappropriate indication

LV Function

LVEF > 40%	0
LVEF < 40%	+

Appropriateness of PCI in ACS Setting

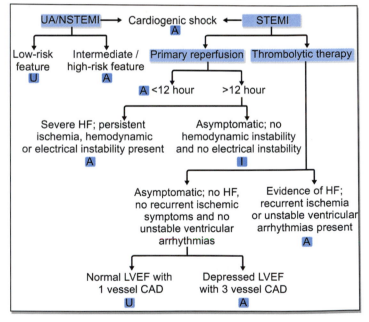

Suggested Reading

1. Chan PS, Brindis RG, Cohen DJ. Concordance of physician rating with appropriate use criteria for coronary revascularization. J Am Coll Cardiol. 2011;57:1546-53.
2. Kappetein AP, Mohr FW, Feldman TF. Comparison of coronary bypass surgery with drug eluting stenting for treatment of left main and/or three vessel disease: 3-year follow-up of the SYNTAX trial. Eur Heart J. 2011;17:2125-34.

3. Ko DT, Guo H, Wijeysundera HC, et al. Assessing the association of appropriateness of coronary revascularization and clinical outcomes for patients with stable coronary artery disease. J Am Coll Cardiol. 2012;60:1876-84.

4. Patel MR, Dehmen GJ, Hirshfeld JW et al. ACCF/SCAI/STS/AATS/AHA/ASNC/HFSA/SCCT. Appropriate use of criteria for coronary revascularization focused update. J Am Coll Cardiol. 2012;59(9):857-81.

5. Sanchez CE, Marroquin O, Lee J, et al. The revascularization Heart Team approach complements appropriate use criteria for coronary revascularization. J Am Coll Cardiol 2014;63:12-5.

2

Percutaneous Coronary Intervention: Work Station
(The Unsung Heroics)

■ Sabyasachi Mitra, Shuvanan Ray

Introduction

Though there is a tendency to rate percutaneous coronary intervention (PCI) to almost a procedure such as sebaceous cyst excision or any outdoor surgery, it is actually not so. It is a procedure which can turn ugly at any moment and can produce severe consequences, even death.

A survey (Institute of Medicine Report, 1999) showed that 44,000–98,000 deaths annually happened from adverse events during procedure which is equivalent to 1 airplane crash each day. Most of the cases were related to either a mistake in picking-up a cue before sending to cathlab or missing out a drug before or during the procedure (like antiplatelets/heparin). Patients and relatives do not understand the heroics in cathlab, but they remember the welcoming environment, prompt professional work-up and a transparent billing related to the procedure, and this requires a team rather than an individual. A dedicated team working with a definite protocol and check-list can significantly reduce morbidity and mortality in patients undergoing any surgical procedures including percutaneous cardiovascular intervention.

Components of Cathlab Team

- Physician [(Primary Operator, PO)]
- *Secondary operators:* Assistant to PO
- Physicians assistants

- *Nurse supervisor:* This person must be familiar with the overall function of the laboratory, have strong management skills, help set tone of patient surroundings and be in charge of preprocedure and postprocedure holding areas. Nurse supervisor should ensure that institutional guidelines for patient monitoring, drug administration, protocols for patient care (including protocols for handling potential complications) are established and that all catheterization laboratory nurses are properly trained.
- *Cathlab nurses:* Background of such nurses should be from critical care experience including knowledge of cardiovascular medications, intravenous (IV) infusion and sterile techniques. Experienced with vascular catheter instrumentation, especially with identification, cleaning, sterilization and storage.
- *Non-nursing personnel:*
  - *Technologist:* Should have proper radiology and angiography training, experience about X-ray generators, cine pulse systems,

image intensification, cine and digital imaging and storage, pressure injection system and radiation safety principles.

– *Additional administrative personnel:*
  » Scheduler/case manager
  » Inventory manager
  » Database or administrative staff
– Billing and customer care officer

1. *Duty of cathlab team—pre-PCI:*
   C : Check (Point by point of a checklist)
   A : Avoid (Offending drugs and adverse lab/hemodynamic irregul-
   arities)
   R : Reset: Blood sugar
   Drugs: [Dual anti-platelets therapy (DAPT), IV fluid, sedation, premedications]
   E : Explain to patient and relatives

2. *Checklist—components:*
   – Patient identification, consent confirmed
   – Patient's recent clinical status/potential complication reviewed [ejection fraction (EF), congestive heart failure (CHF), shock]
   – Procedure, indication
   – Equipment needed available
   – Access site planned
   – Allergies (especially contrast) and premedications
   – Antibiotic prophylaxis for implants
   – Labs reviewed

3. *Most important laboratory reports:*
   – Hb%, hematocrit (>30/stable)
   – Potassium—3.5–5 mEq/L.
   – Creatinine/BUN/albumin
   – International normalized ratio (INR)
   – Platelets > 50,000/dL
   – Serology

4. *Calculations:*
   – eGFR (MDRD)
   – Bleeding score
   – Overall mortality score
   – Syntax score.

Estimated Glomerular Filtration Rate Calculation and Prevention of Contrast-induced Nephropathy

The development of contrast-induced nephropathy (CIN) also referred to as contrast-induced acute kidney injury, is a significant complication of intravascular contrast medium, use of which is linked with excessive morbidity and mortality. Although the serum level of creatinine is widely used in the diagnosis of renal impairment in CIN, the serum level is an unreliable indicator of kidney function because creatinine is not a real time biomarker. Both glomerular filtration rate (GFR) and creatinine clearance reflect filtration of creatinine. However GFR is considered a more accurate index of kidney function. GFR provides a more accurate account of working nephrons that is based on glomerular filtration. The National Kidney Foundation Kidney Disease Outcome Quality Initiative recommends that clinicians

Table 2.1: Cardiovascular research foundation risk score for CIN

Risk factors	Integer score
Hypotension	5
Intra-aortic balloon pump (IABP)	5
Congestive heart failure (CHF)	5
Age > 75 years	4
Anemia	3
Diabetes	3
Contrast media volume	1

Serum creatinine > 1.5 mg/dL : 4
or
eGFR < 60 mL/min/1.73 m² : 2 → 40–60
4 → 20–40
6 → <20

Risk score	Risk of CIN	Risk of dialysis
≤5	7.5%	0.04%
6–0	14%	0.12%
11–16	26.1%	1.09%
>16	57.3%	12.6%

should use estimated GFR (eGFR) calculated on the basis of the serum level of creatinine. Patients with a GFR < 60 mL/min/1.73 m² have considerable loss of nephron units.

Risk score for CIN: In an attempt to provide an aid towards a rapid bedside identification of patients at increased risk for CIN, several risk prediction tools have been recently developed which can be used also for institution of quality improvement interventions aimed toward the reduction of contrast nephropathy and nephropathy requiring dialysis, in such patients (Table 2.1).

Calculation

- Percent risk of CIN can be roughly calculated by multiplying serum creatinine concentration in milligrams per deciliter by 10
- *Volume of contrast media:* Some studies found a correlation between the volume of contrast given and the risk of nephropathy. The limit was 5 mL of contrast per kg body weight up to a maximum of 300 mL divided by serum creatinine concentration in mg/dL. Nephropathy developed in 21% of the patients in whom the total volume of contrast exceeded the formula amount, compared with 2% (P < 0.001) of patients in whom the contrast volume fell within the prescribed limit.
- *Types of contrast media:* Low osmolar agents reduces the incidence of CIN in comparison to high osmolar agents. So low osmolar agents (Iohexol, Ioxaglate—Osmolality 600–900 moSm/L) are used frequently. The newest agent is isosmolar (Iodixanole, 300 moSm/L). It was seen to reduce the incidence of CIN in high-risk patients but larger RCTs are needed to verify this encouraging result.

Prevention (Flow Chart 2.1)

- Avoid dehydration
- Contrast volume and frequency of administration should be minimized. Avoid repeat injection within 72 hours.
- Low osmolar/isosmolar contrast
- Nephrotoxic drugs to be discontinued 48 prior to contrast injection (Metformin, ACEI, ARB, NSAIDs, aminoglycosides).

Hydration: The experimental and clinical studies support the use of intravenous hydration to prevent CIN, especially in patients with azotemia at high risk. Intravenous sodium chloride 1 mL/kg/hour (max 100 mL/hour) 12 hours pre- and 12 hours postcontrast (24 hours total infusion duration) can be given as a protocol in every patient who needs intervention. If there is CHF or low left ventricular ejection fraction (LVEF <40%) IV fluid should be infused 0.5 mL/kg/hour (maximum 50 mL/hour) 12 hours pre- and postcontrast (24 hours total infusion duration).

In emergency procedure—0.9% NS: 3 mL/kg/hour bolus infusion 1 hour before contrast administration followed by an infusion of 1.5 mL/kg/hour during the procedure and for 4 hours thereafter.

Sodium Bicarbonate Preparation

Sodium bicarbonate in some small studies has been observed to reduce incidence to CIN compared to NS. Add 6.5 amps of 7.5% w/v sodium bicarbonate (150 mEq) in 1 liter of 5% distilled water 3 mL/kg/hour of this solution for 1 hour before contrast administration and then for 6 hours afterward (In diabetics, mixing sodium bicarbonate in 1 liter of sterile water).

N acetylcysteine: Its value in preventing CIN is controversial.
Dose—N Acetylcysteine
- 600–1200 mg capsules PO every 12 hours × 4 doses.
  2 doses precontrast and 2 doses postcontrast is optimal.
- Emergent procedure
  1 dose before and 3 doses postcath or procedure is acceptable (every 12 hours × 4 doses total).

Flow chart 2.1: Prevention of contrast-induced nephropathy

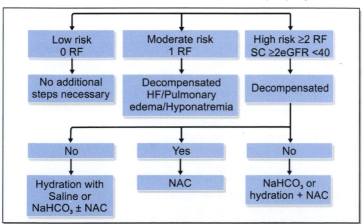

Hemodialysis and Hemofiltration

Most people can safely wait 24–36 hours after contrast exposure until next hemodialysis treatment.

Bleeding

Bleeding is the most common complication following PCI and is associated with an increased risk of other adverse outcomes. Bleeding was defined as occurring at percutaneous entry site, during or after catheterization laboratory visit until discharge, which may be external or a hematoma > 10 cm for femoral, > 5 cm for brachial or > 2 cm for radial access or retroperitoneal or gastrointestinal or genitourinary or/other unknown origin during or after catheterization until discharge and required a transfusion, prolonged hospital stay and/or a drop of hemoglobin > 3.0 g/dL (NCDR, Cath PCI data).

There are other definitions of bleeding in PCI (Table 2.2).

Bleeding Scores

National Cardiovascular Data Registry (NCDR) data has derived a bleeding score to predict bleeding after PCI which includes both acute and chronic cases (i.e. in ACS or chronic stable patients), whereas there are others which predict bleeding in acute situations or after use of specific agents. A bleeding score calculation is necessary to calculate the bleeding risk and to use agents during PCI accordingly to avoid post-PCI bleeding which is correlated with increased mortality (Table 2.3 and Fig. 2.1).

Strategies to Reduce Bleeding Risk

- *ACT to desired level:* ACT should be kept between 200 and 250, if GPIIbIIIa inhibitors are used, otherwise between 250 and 300, if it is not used. ACT above 350 has not only been demonstrated to increase the risk of bleeding, but also increase the ischemic complications such as myocardial infarction, death or revascularization.
- Addition of GPIIb/IIIa inhibitors with unfractionated heparin (UFH) increases the risk of access site bleeding in patients with high bleeding score. It seems reasonable that appropriate dosing of antithrombotic agents based on weight and renal clearance is an important step to reduce bleeding risk.

Table 2.2: TIMI bleeding definitions

Major	ICH
	≥ 5 g/dL, decrease in Hb% conc.
	≥ 15% absolute decrease in hematocrit
Minor	Observed blood loss
	≥ 3 g/dL decrease in Hb% conc.
	≥ 10% decrease in the hematocrit
	No-observed blood loss
	≥ 4 g/dL decrease in Hb% conc.
	≥ 12% decrease in the hematocrit
Minimal	Any clinically overt sign of hemorrhage associated with a
	< 3 g/dL decrease in Hb% conc. or
	< 9% decrease in hematocrit

Table 2.3: NCDR Cath PCI bleeding risk score

Variable	Score			
STEMI	No	Yes		
	0	15		
Age (years)	<60	60–70	71–79	>80
	0	10	15	20
BMI	<20	20–30	31–9	>40
	15	5	0	5
Previous PCI	No	Yes		
	10	0		
Chronic kidney disease	No	Mild	Moderate	Dialysis
	0	10	25	30
Shock	No	Yes		
	0	35		
Cardiac arrest < 24 hours	No	Yes		
	0	15		
Female	No	Yes		
	0	20		
Hemoglobin	<13	13–15	>15	
	5	0	10	
PCI Status	Elective	Urgent	Emergency/ salvage	
	0	20	40	

(NCDR, National Cardiovascular Data Registry)

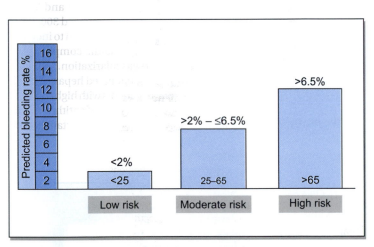

Fig. 2.1: Risk of post-PCI bleeding

- Bivalirudin was shown to reduce bleeding in the earlier trials, but has shown to increase acute stent thrombosis in recent trials. Its use is debated but in high bleeding score patients, it still remains a choice.
- Change of access from femoral to radial in high bleeding score patients may help.

SYNTAX and Clinical SYNTAX Score

Syntax score is a well-established angiographic tool to predict long-term outcomes after PCI (Chapter 5, pg 62). The logistic clinical syntax score has been shown to perform better than syntax score alone in predicting 1 year outcomes, and even 3 years outcomes after PCI (Table 2.4 and Fig. 2.2).

Clinical SYNTAX Score

Low   :   <8
Medium :   8–17
High   :   >17

A Few Words About Consent

Informed consent is most often viewed by interventional cardiologist as a legal obligation that must be fulfilled in order to perform the procedure requested but actually physician must understand that:
1. It is a serious legal obligation inextricably linked to physicians ethical obligations to his/her patient
2. It represents an important opportunity for managing risk.

What is an informed consent?
It is not simply securing a signature on a consent form. It is the education of the patient that should occur in conversation between physician and the patient in which the patient obtains sufficient information to make a knowing decision.

Table 2.4: Clinical SYNTAX score

Extended model	Score				
SYNTAX score	≤17	17–32	>33		
	0	1	2		
Age in years	<50	50–59	60–69	70–79	>80
	0	2	4	6	8
Creatinine clearance	<30	30–59	60–89	>90	
(mL/min)	6	4	2	0	
LVEF	<30	30–39	40–49	>50	
	6	4	2	0	
SYNTAX like patient	No	Yes			
(LMCA/3VD)	0	2			
BMI	<20	21–29	30–34	35–39	>40
	1	0	1	2	3
Diabetes mellitus	No	Yes			
	0	2			
Peripheral vascular disease	No	Yes			
	0	3			

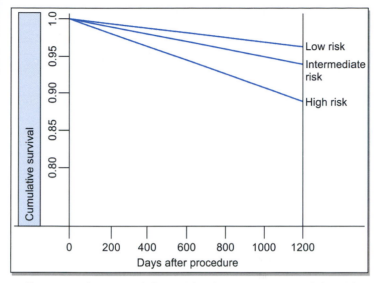

Fig. 2.2: Cumulative survival after PCI (Clinical SYNTAX Score): Extended model

This should include the proposed treatment and alternatives, risks and benefits and should culminate in an agreement obtained from informed patient.

Who should obtain the consent?
It is a nondelegable duty of the primary physician proposing the therapy.

When it should be obtained?
It should not be taken on the operating table or cathlab. Ideally, a consent should be taken when the patient is comfortable, not sedated and free to listen and capable of taking decisions.

What a consent form should contain?
- The nature of the patient's condition, illness or diagnosis
- The proposed treatment plan
- The risks, side effects and complications (those which are most commonly associated)
- A description of the risks and benefits of the reasonable alternatives to the proposed treatment plan (including the alternative on non-treatment)
- A record of any brochures or other written or audiovisual information relating to the procedure given to the patient
- That the patient had an opportunity to ask questions and that those questions were answered to his or her satisfaction before signing the form
- Along with the printed consent, the specific points of discussions and agreement should be written by the primary physician and that should be supported by the patient in his/her own language and handwriting.

Diabetic Patients before PCI

- *Glycemic target:* Between 140 and 200 mg/dL.
  For patients who are eating (most of the PCI patients), we aim for a fasting glucose of <140 mg/dL. with random glucose level < 180 mg/dL.

Table 2.5: Commonly used insulins

Insulin type	Onset	Peak	Duration
Lispro aspart	5–15 min	45–75 min	2–4 hour
Regular	about 30 min	2–4 hour	5–8 hour
NPH	about 2 hour	4–12 hour	18–28 hour
Insulin glargine	about 2 hour	No peak	20–> 24 hour
Insulin detemir	about 2 hour	3–9 hour	6–24 hour
NPL	about 2 hour	6 hour	15 hour
Insulin degludec	about 2 hour	No peak	> 40 hour

Table 2.6: Subcutaneous sliding scale using short-acting insulins

Glucose values (mg/dL)	Insulin sensitive		Normal		Insulin resistant	
	AC	HS	AC	HS	AC	HS
< 150	0	0	0	0	0	0
151–200	0	0	2	0	4	2
201–250	2	0	4	0	8	4
251–300	3	1	6	2	12	6
301–350	4	2	8	4	16	8
351–400	5	3	10	6	20	10

AC: Before meal; HS: Bed time

- It is better to hold oral hypoglycemic drugs or noninsulin injectables (exenatide/Liraglutides—GLP-1 analogs) in the morning of the procedure. For patients who develop hyperglycemia, supplemental short or rapid acting insulin may be administered subcutaneously (typically, every 6 hours) (Table 2.5) based on frequently (every 1–2 hours) measured glucose levels which are often obtained on capillary fingerstick samples (Table 2.6).

Correction insulin: Varying doses of short or rapid-acting insulin can be added to usual premeal short or rapid-acting insulin in patients with basal bolus insulin requirements to correct premeal glucose excursions. This is called correction insulin.

Typically given when glucose levels are > 150 mg/dL.

- *Insulin sensitive:* Older, T-1 diabetes mellitus, chronic kidney disease, chronic liver disease.
- *Insulin resistant:* Obesity, patients on glucocorticoids.
- Those patients who take insulin (intermediate or long and rapid or short acting) only in the morning should be given half or one-third of their total morning dose of insulin as intermediate, or long-acting insulin to provide basal insulin conc. during the procedure and prevent ketosis.
- For patients, who take mixed dose (intermediate/long and rapid/short) two or more times per day, should be given one-third to one half of the total morning dose (both types) as intermediate or long acting.

- Patients on continuous insulin infusion (pump) continue with their usual basal infusion rates.
- A dextrose containing IV solution (mixture of 5% dextrose and 0.45% normal saline) should be started at the rate of 75–125 mL/hour to provide 3.75–6.25 g of glucose/hour to avoid metabolic changes of starvation.
- Blood sugar by finger stick should be checked (or by laboratory method—if critically ill) every hour and more frequently, if blood glucose is < 100 mg/dL, or if the rate of fall is rapid.
- For patients who develop hyperglycemia, supplemental short- or rapid-acting insulin may be administered subcutaneously based on frequently measured glucose levels by fingerstick method (correction insulin).

Postprocedure Care

Arterial and venous sheaths (introducers) are small flexible catheters, used as a guide for wires, stents, balloons, rotoblades, etc. that are passed through the sheath to perform diagnostic procedures and percutaneous interventions (PCI's)

Once the procedure in cathlab has been completed, the sheath remains in place for (in general), a short period of time before removal.

Sheath removal for percutaneous coronary interventions (PCIs) generally occurs outside of the cathlab; optimal time for removal postprocedure varies according to procedure and the activated clotting time (ACT) is usually below 180.

Postoperative ward should have a very important checklist, which should be maintained with utmost care and dedication. A model checklist may be as follows:

Postcath Checklist

Receive a patient
- *Symptoms:* Note, if any
- *Hemodynamics:*
  - Heart rate
  - Blood pressure
  - Respiratory rate
  - SpO_2
- *Groin* (In case of femoral access):
  - Hematoma (if any, mark the boundary with a marker pen)
  - Bleeding
  - Measure the thigh with a measuring tape at a fixed distance from a fixed point (e.g. ASIS/lateral trochanter) and note
- *Lungs:* Crepts, if any
  - Basal
  - Mid
  - Apex
- *IV lines:*
  - Fluid direction [........ mL/kg/hour]
  - Drugs [if any, check and note]
- *Urine volume:* In high risk, hemodynamically unstable patients, urinary Foley's catheter for hourly urine volume

- Capillary blood glucose
- Check oral drugs
- *Position of patient:* Patient should be kept in supine position. A position greater than 20° semi-Fowler's position could lead to flexing and kinking of the femoral sheath resulting in clot formation and possible thrombus.

Check all those parameters every 15 minutes for 4 hours
    Send for ACT after 4 hours, if < 180, remove sheath
**Check all parameters after sheath removal*
    Every 15 minutes for 4 hours
    Every 30 minutes for 8 hours
    Every 60 minutes for 8 hours

Premedications Before Sheath Removal

Premedication with atropine, sedatives, analgesia, and fluid bolus will assist in the prevention of a vasovagal episode that may be induced by the pain of manual/mechanical pressure.

- *Atropine* 0.6 mg direct IV.
- *Midazolam* 1 mg direct IV to sedate and help prevent a vasovagal episode. (Alternatively, diazepam 2.5–10 mg is used somewhere).
- *Lignocaine* (10–20 mL) as a local infiltration around the sheath site, to reduce pain during compression.
- *IV bolus 200 mL* of normal saline.
- Pain medication as ordered to prevent vasovagal episode and possibly reduce the amount of sedation needed.

IV Direct Atropine

- Following the administration of atropine, the nurse will continue to monitor for drug effects; radial pulse is assessed every 5 minutes × 2.
- Do not administer atropine, if the pulse is greater than 100/min. Notify the physician immediately, if the pulse is greater than 120/minute following administration and the patient is symptomatic or complaining of chest pain (Excessive cardioacceleration can precipitate or *worsen arrhythmias or ischemia or increase degree of infarction).*

Midazolam/Diazepam

- When deciding the dose, consider the patient's age, weight, anxiety level and response to recent administration of pain medications.
- To prevent inadvertent oversedation, begin with a smaller dose and administer additional sedation according to the patient's response/need throughout the procedure.
- Obtain baseline pulse, respiratory rate and O_2 saturation level prior to administration.
- Continue to monitor until groin compression is complete and hemostasis achieved.
- Notify the physician, if O_2 saturation is less than or equal to 90% or where rapid desaturation from baseline is noted.
- Suction, O_2 and antidote/reversal agent for sedation must be readily available on the unit

Access care: Currently, three main techniques are used to achieve hemostasis in the femoral access site after PCI. Manual compression, mechanical compression, vascular closure:

1. *Manual compression:* Manual compression has been the gold standard for obtaining hemostasis at the vascular access site for years, but the standard has changed as new devices have been introduced. Pressure is applied as the sheath is removed by placing the index and the middle fingers 1–2 cm above the site where the sheath enters the skin and applying pressure as the sheath is removed. Hemostasis is achieved by compressing the femoral artery against femoral head.

    • Manual compression requires strength and ability to hold a good compression for 15–20 minutes. If hand and arm fatigue develops during the procedure, the amount of pressure applied to the femoral artery may vary leading to vascular access site complications.

2. *Mechanical compression:* Mechanical compression involves the application of constant pressure in the artery to obtain hemostasis and allows hands-free catheter removal so that patient can be better monitored. There are two main types of compressions:

    i. *C Clamp (Compress AR, Advance Vascular Dynamics):* It consists of a flat metal plate placed under the mattress at the patient's hip to stabilize the device and a C Clamp arm. A disposable translucent pad is attached to the tip of the C Clamp arm. The translucent pad is placed 1–2 cm above the site, where the sheath enters the skin and pressure is applied by pressing down on the C Clamp arm.

    ii. *The Femostop device (Radi Medical Systems AB, St Jude Medical Inc.):* This device uses a small pneumatic clear pressure dome, a belt placed around the patient's hip and a pump and a manometer making it possible to adjust pressure to an optimum level.

    The time from application to removal of compression devices should ideally be less than 30 minutes.

3. *Vascular closure devices:* These devices first appeared in the 1990s as means of reducing time on bed rest and improving both hemostasis and patient's comfort. A variety of devices seek to mechanically close the arterial puncture site during sheath removal in the catheterization laboratory in fully anticoagulated patients and shorten the time of hemostasis and ambulation. Three main types of vascular closure devices can be categorized by mechanism of hemostasis, including sutures (Perclose—Abbott Vascular), collagen-like plugs (Angioseal–Radi Medical Systems AB) and staples/clips (Starclose—Abbott Vascular). Suture-mediated closure devices tie-off the femoral artery with sutures.

    Collagen plugs seal the puncture site by stimulating platelet aggregation and the release of coagulation factors which results in the formation of a clot.

    Extravascular clips or staples are used to seal the puncture site in the artery. Hemostasis is obtained shortly after deployment allowing the patient to get out of the bed and ambulate faster.

    Few important words about VCD:

    • Patient should be selected properly
    • To be used in patients after PCI with high bleeding risk, e.g.
        a. Obese patients
        b. Low puncture but not involving the bifurcation of CFA
    • They should not be used in presence of peripheral vascular disease involving femoral arteries.

Procedure of Sheath Removal

- The patient is assisted to move closer to the side of the bed and positioned so that the arterial clamp can be applied, if needed.
- The patient is then pre-medicated.
- The occlusive dressing is carefully removed from the sheath
- Generally, the left hand is used to compress the right femoral artery, while the right hand is used to compress the left femoral artery.
- Manual pressure is applied to the artery so that the index finger is placed on the site where the sheath enters the femoral artery.
- The middle and ring fingers of the same hand are used to reinforce compression.
- After the hand is placed on the artery, manual pressure is applied as the arterial sheath is gently removed from the site.
- Just enough pressure is applied to avoid excessive blood loss; however, a small amount of blood should be allowed to escape from the artery in case of thrombus formation associated within the sheath.
- After allowing a small amount of blood to escape, firm pressure is applied. Apply just enough pressure to achieve hemostasis *but not obliterate the pedal pulses.*
- Expect the pulses to be diminished. An assistant can determine by Doppler the presence of the pedal pulse prior to compression and the diminution of the pedal pulse when sufficient pressure has been applied to the femoral artery.
- Maintain this pressure level for a period of 3–5 minutes.
- Gradually release the pressure to allow the pedal pulse to progressively strengthen. Maintain a delay between when the pulse is felt by the compressing hand and when it is felt by the hand palpating the pedal pulse. Maintain this amount of pressure for another five minutes.
- The pressure is gradually removed over 5–10 minutes allowing for a progressive strengthening of the pedal pulse.
- With the non-compressing hand, palpate the femoral area around the compressing hand to ensure there is no occult hematoma formation.
- If there is evidence of bleeding from the puncture site or increasing hematoma formation as pressure is released from the femoral artery, apply more pressure to the artery.
- When applying manual pressure, remove the venous sheath 5–10 minutes *after* pulling the arterial sheath as long as control of arterial bleeding has been achieved manually or with the groin clamp. If despite 15–20 minutes of manual pressure, then there is bleeding or continuing hematoma formation, then the clamp should be applied.

Concurrent removal of both venous and arterial sheath should be avoided as:
- Removing both sheaths at the same time increases the risk of arteriovenous fistula formation.
- Compress above and below the sheath entrance as the sheath is gently removed.
- Maintain firm pressure for five minutes.

- If desired, venous sheath removal may be delayed until complete control of arterial bleeding has been achieved (manual/clamp pressure has been removed with no evidence of bleeding).
- Prolonged pressure on the femoral vein should be avoided.
- Although rare, prolonged venous occlusion, especially where a clamp is used, may lead to venous thrombosis.
- Leg/foot cyanosis, pain and swelling of the affected limb could be an indication of venous thrombosis and should be reported immediately.

Access Site Care: Radial Artery

- Radial sheath is removed just after the procedure, on full anticoagulation, in the cathlab.
- Post-procedure, while transradial band is on, check wrist every 15 minutes for bleeding, hematoma, capillary refilling, color warmth, and pulse oximetry.
- Start to deflate in 2 hours following diagnostic procedure.
- Start to deflate in 4 hours following any intervention.
- Once off, check site every 15 minutes for the 1st hour, then every 30 minutes for the next hour, and then every hour for the next 2 hours.

Radial Access Closure alternative to Radial Band

- Cut elastic adhesive bandage (2 inch) × (4–6 inch) × 3 such
- Place the strips over the procedure site (covered by a small cotton wool) (Fig. 2.3)
- Place additional strip, if necessary, above or below.

Radial Hematoma (Fig. 2.4)

- Notify the physician/Interventional cardiologist
- Can follow forearm diameter and keep records
- Place additional band above or below the initial band
- Inflate blood pressure Cuff to < 20 mm of Hg of the systolic blood pressure of the patient, if Grade III/IV hematoma is seen. Deflate the cuff, every 15 minutes.
  - Can also place the pulse oxymeter on the finger in the same arm, to ensure presence of waveform.
- Place icebag or cold compress on the hematoma.

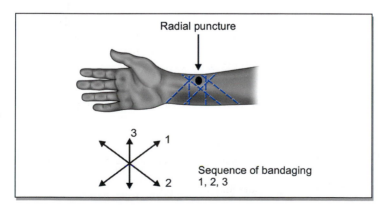

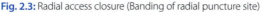

Fig. 2.3: Radial access closure (Banding of radial puncture site)

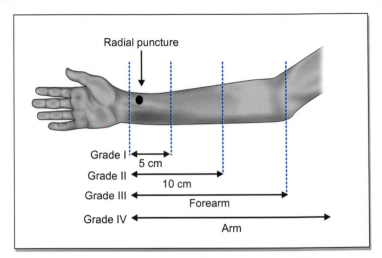

Fig. 2.4: EASY hematoma classification after transradial PCI (EASY, Embolism Assessment of Safety and Efficacy)

Potential Complications of Sheath Removal and Necessary Actions

Excess Blood Return Around the Sheath

- Notify interventional cardiologist, while applying pressure dressing to groin area.
- Assist in insertion of larger sheath, if necessary.
- Consult physician regarding stopping heparin, measuring ACT and early sheath removal, if appropriate.

Vasovagal Episode

- Take steps to prevent vasovagal episode
- Give IV bolus 200–500 mL normal saline, atropine 0.6 mg direct IV, sedation with IV midazolam 1 mg, Lignocaine (10–20 mL) local infiltration prior to sheath removal.
- Recognize symptoms.
- Reapply manual pressure, if necessary.
- Check vital signs every 5 minutes until they return to prevasovagal episode level.
- If no response, ask physician to assess.

Chest Pain

- Obtain description of pain and record vital signs.
- Obtain 12 lead ECG.
- Treat with O_2 and nitroglycerin 0.3–0.6 mg every 5 minutes × 3.
- If no response, notify interventional cardiologist.

Bleeding or Hematoma

- Reapply manual pressure to femoral artery × 10–15 minutes.
- Apply clamp, if manual pressure not effective.
- Observe patient for vasovagal episode and treat, if necessary.
- Contact physician, if still unable to control bleeding.

Retroperitoneal Bleeding

- Recognize signs and symptoms—moderate—severe pain in the back, flank, leg, lower abdominal quadrant or groin along with tachycardia and hypotension.
- Notify physician.

Pseudoaneurysm/AV Fistula

- Assess for symptoms, which include pulsatile, usually painful mass over the artery at the puncture site and possible nerve compression by the mass resulting in sharp, stabbing or shooting pain in the groin which may radiate down the thigh.
- Auscultate for femoral bruit and notify physician, if present.

Arterial Occlusion

- Allow a small amount of blood to escape prior to compressing the artery to expel any clots
- Know the signs and symptoms—may include sudden onset of severe pain or numbness, pallor, cyanosis or absence of distal pulses in the affected limb.
- Notify physician.

Infection

- Know signs and symptoms, and educate patient about swelling, redness, warm skin and purulent drainage at the insertion site.
- Notify physician.

Neuropathy

- Know signs and symptoms—may include pain, tingling at groin site, numbness at site or down leg, motor difficulty with affected leg, possible decreased patellar tendon reflex and possible weakness of knee extension. Symptoms may occur as long as three months after the procedure.
- Notify physician.

Femoral Pseudoaneurysm (Fig. 2.5)

Duplex scanning was performed in patients who were suspected of having local groin vascular complications based on the presence of one or more of the following at the puncture site:

- Pain
- Extensive skin discoloration or ecchymosis
- Palpable or pulsatile mass
- Thrill or bruit

The following parameters were reported during scanning in cases with fulfilled duplex criteria of femoral pseudoaneurysm:

- Echolucent sac that expands and contracts with each cardiac contraction.
- Color Doppler showing swirling flow pattern with turbulence in the sac with a track connection with the femoral artery.
- When a pulsed-wave Doppler is placed in the neck, a 'to and fro' signal is obtained, which signifies that this is in fact a pseudoaneurysm.

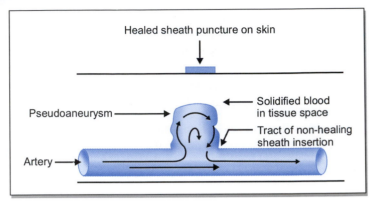

Fig. 2.5: Femoral psuedoaneurysm

Events After Percutaneous Coronary Intervention

Remember CVPN

- *Cardiac:* Ischemia/infarction, tamponade, arrhythmia including ventricular tachycardia, heart block, bradycardia, coronary artery perforation, coronary artery dissection, air embolism.
- *Vascular:* Aortic dissection, access site complications, distal embolization
- *Pulmonary:* Pulmonary edema due to congestive heart failure, or large contrast load, anaphylaxis
- *Neurologic:* Stroke due to atheromatous/air embolization, sedative effect, global ischemia and hypoxia from shock.

To be watched carefully:
- *Chest pain:* Chest pain occurs in 50% of the patients after PCI and chest pain may be benign or may be a sign of a grave prognosis (Table 2.7 and Flow chart 2.2).
- *Hypotension:* Not a very uncommon complication after PCI. Reasons are:
  – Acute vessel closure
  – Coronary perforation/tamponade
  – Hypovolemia/bleeding
  – Vagal reaction
  – Drug reaction
  – Dissection of coronary arteries.

Table 2.7: Reasons of chest pain

- Benign stent sensation
- Acute stent thrombosis
- Abrupt vessel closure
- Transient coronary spasm
- Side branch occlusion
- Distal embolization of debris

All chest pain should be reported to the physician and ECG (12 leads) should be done as, and when necessary.

Flow chart 2.2: Chest pain algorithm

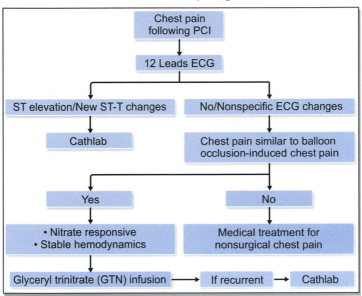

Flow chart 2.3: Algorithm for post-PCI hypotension

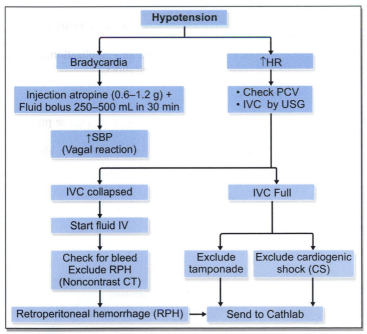

Hypotension is defined as systolic BP (SBP) < 90 mm Hg or SBP 30 mm lower than patient's entrance BP. Any SBP < 90 mm Hg needs attention, regardless the starting point.

Most common is vagal reaction due to combination of back pain (pre-existing or possibly new) related to the required recumbent positioning during or after the procedure and groin puncture site pain (sometimes from the compression). The treatment is to give 250–500 cc NS over 20–30 minutes, atropine 0.5 mg IV and some mild analgesia may be used, like low dose fentanyl (12.5 mg) IV. In elderly, the vagal reaction may not manifest bradycardia. Restoration of the SBP should validate that this initial episode of hypotension was likely vagal.

Next most common cause of hypotension would be that of volume loss; i.e. bleeding. Bleeding from the vascular access site is responsible about 90% of the time, but spontaneous bleeding away from access site can also occur.

Other causes include cardiac tamponade and acute ischemic complications (Flow chart 2.3).

Suggested Reading

1. Expert consensus document on cardiac catheterization – Laboratory standard update (A CC/SCA I – 2012. J Am Coll Cardiol. 2013;59:24:2012-221.
2. Haynes AB, Berry WR. A surgical safety checklist to reduce morbidity and mortality in global population. NEJM. 2009;5:360.
3. Iqbal J. Predicting 3 year mortality after PCI. J Am Coll Cardiol Intervention. 2014;7:5:13-8.
4. Mauro Moscucci. Complications of Cardiovascular Procedures. Wolter Kluwer/Lippincott Williams & Wilkins, 2011.
5. Meliran Roxana. A simple risk score for prediction of contrast induced nephropathy after PCI. J Am Coll Cardiol. 2004;44:1393-9.
6. Vavalle JP. Interv Cardiol. 2009;1(I):51-62.

3

Access
(The Gateway of PCI)

- Shuvanan Ray

Percutaneous Seldinger technique changed the choice of access for percutaneous coronary intervention (PCI) to femoral artery, and it became a rule. Later, radial artery and occasionally, ulnar arteries are being used, and particularly radial access is getting such popularity that it has become a parallel institution.

Why Radial Access?

Problems of radial access: Radial access has some problems which can be overcome with practice.

- More muscular artery which has a tendency to develop spasm, producing pain and difficulty in catheter manipulation. This can happen in spite of drugs to combat.
- Anatomical variations, severe tortuosities or loops in radial or brachial arteries (incidence is close to 5%).
- Access does not allow catheters > 7F.
- Back-up support may be under question in some complex procedures.

So access for PCI is mostly femoral and radial; and a budding interventional cardiologist must know at least these two accesses thoroughly (Table 3.1).

Femoral Access

For femoral access, few important points are to be remembered:

- Puncture should be done in the common femoral artery.
- It must be an anterior wall puncture.

Table 3.1: Advantages of radial access: Less access-related complications compared to femoral

Complications	Femoral (%)	Radial (%)
Hematoma (>5–10 mL)	<5	1–3
Retroperitoneal bleeding	<2	0
Pseudoaneurysm	1–2	<0.1
AV fistula	1–2	<0.8
Limb ischemia	<0.1	Extremely rare
Infection	<5	<0.1
Dissection/Perforation	<1	<1

How You Locate the Common Femoral Artery (Fig. 3.1)?

- Skin crease and inguinal ligament by surface marking
- Radiological marker—the femoral head
- Arterial calcification, if any
- USG-guided puncture

Femoral access is not a very difficult procedure to learn, particularly in a young, non-obese, male subject, but it is difficult and needs attention and planning in obese, female and elderly patients.

- *Inguinal ligament* is the most important surface marking for femoral access, because it is the line at which the 'u'-shaped origin of inferior epigastric artery takes place, and any puncture at or above the site would cause damage to the artery leading to retroperitoneal hemorrhage. So upper limit of the puncture must be the inguinal ligament.
- *Skin crease and inguinal ligament:* It is to be stressed that inguinal skin crease does not corroborate with inguinal ligament, particularly in obese patients or patients with lax abdominal wall.
- *Radiological marker:* It is seen that the radiological marker for perfect femoral puncture is the midpoint of femoral head. The common femoral artery (CFA) extends along the length of femoral head. So to locate the puncture site, it is better to locate femoral head in AP view with leg externally rotated and knee extended. A metal hemostat is used as a marker to identify the best location of femoral artery cannulation. This is achieved by a skin puncture done at the lower border of femoral head with the needle entering the skin at 30–45° angle (steeper angle in more obese patient).

  It is not advisable to puncture lower (near or below femoral head) for the fear of puncturing profunda femoris artery, which gives rise to more pseudoaneurysm formation.
- *USG-guided puncture :* FAUST trial has demonstrated the superiority of USG-guided puncture of CFA in reduction of complications (like major bleeding, retroperitoneal hemorrhage and pseudoaneurysm) over fluoroscopy-guided femoral puncture. Although, it may be beneficial in selected high-risk populations, particularly obese patient on high anticoagulant milieu (like in rescue PCI); USG-guided puncture in all patients cannot be recommended as mandatory.

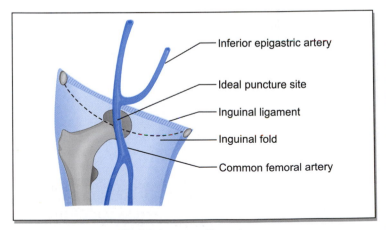

Inferior epigastric artery

Ideal puncture site

Inguinal ligament

Inguinal fold

Common femoral artery

Fig. 3.1: Anatomy of femoral artery

Ultrasound-guided Femoral Puncture

Retrograde Puncture (Fig. 3.2)

- A linear array probe is normally used; this produces a rectangular image, which is displayed with the skin surface at the top, the vertical axis showing depth into the body and the horizontal axis showing position along the probe. When imaging blood vessels, the probe can either be placed along the vessel to produce a longitudinal scan or across the vessel to produce a transverse scan.
- For retrograde femoral puncture, transverse scan is sufficient. But, for antegrade puncture, longitudinal scan helps in directing the wire into SFA.
- Vascular probe just below the inguinal crease with indicator at 9 am direction.
- Femoral artery is located in the middle as pulsatile round shadow; medial to it is elliptical femoral vein which is compressible.
- Needle is inserted just behind the probe to go proximally and it is seen above the femoral arterial shadow—if the needle is pushed, it enters the artery (Fig. 3.3).

Antegrade Puncture

First locate the bifurcation of the femoral artery; once the bifurcation is identified, trace the artery proximally to identify CFA, and then make a transverse scan and try to puncture (Fig. 3.4).

Popliteal access: May be punctured in probe position but we prefer supine puncture.

The patient remains supine with the lower extremity in a 60° externally rotated, and knee in gentle flexion. The puncture site is usually 8–10 cm below the border of the medial condyle of the femur and parallel with the posterior medial border of the tibia for 1 cm. Puncture is performed with 21-gauge needle and a 0.018 inch V-18 guidewire (Boston) (Fig. 3.5).

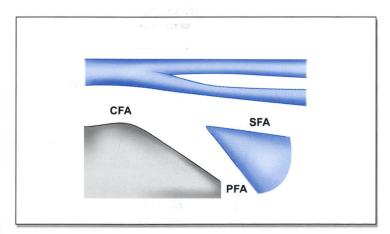

Fig. 3.2: Longitudinal scan of the femoral artery. CFA divides into SFA and PFA. Skin surface is at the top of the image. Arterial blood flow is from left to right

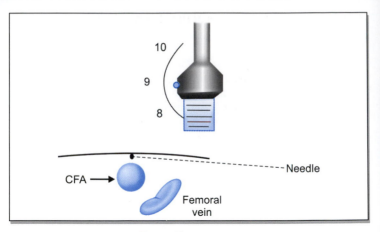

Fig. 3.3: Transverse scan

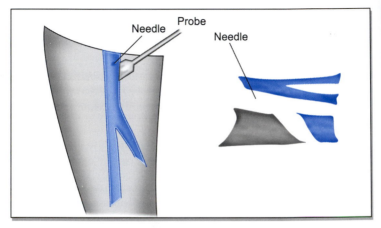

Fig. 3.4: Antegrade femoral puncture

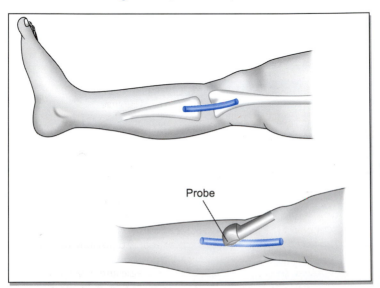

Fig. 3.5: *Popliteal puncture:* Place the vascular probe on popliteal artery and puncture. Leg is slightly flexed at hip and externally rotated at hip

Puncture of Dorsalis Pedis Artery (USG-guided)
(Figs 3.6 and 3.7).

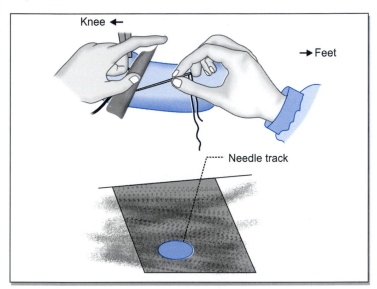

Fig. 3.6: Puncture of Dorsalis pedis artery

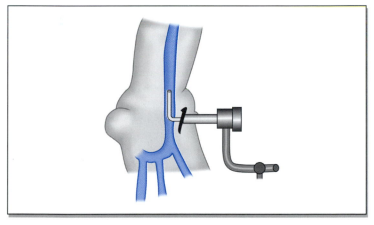

Fig. 3.7: 4F sheath. Dorsalis pedis puncture

How to Perform a Proper Puncture (Fig. 3.8)?

- Locate the puncture site.
- Surface marking of inguinal ligament and 2 cm below it, where maximum pulsation of FA felt; correlate radiologically.
- Feel the pulse with the flat of your fingers (do not buckle).
- With 25-gauge needle, skin is to be infiltrated with 1% lidocaine 2–3 cm below the index finger placed over the artery.
- 10 mL lidocaine is to be given to the skin and possible track of the needle through the subcutaneous tissue.
- Now take a standard arterial puncture needle and place the needle at the site where local anesthetic is given and push the needle at an angle which allows the needle to reach the estimated puncture site on the artery; usually, it is 30–45%.

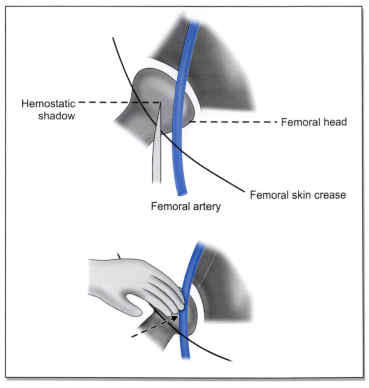

Fig. 3.8: Performing a proper puncture

- When the needle reaches the artery—arterial pulsation can be felt, push the needle a little, the blood jet will come out and anterior puncture of femoral artery is established.
- Put the guidewire through the needle hub. It will be easy to steer till the end.
- Come out with the needle, make a small nick around the wire with 11-blade scalpel.
  Push the sheath in:

> - If the guidewire does not go easily, rotate and manipulate the needle and try to negotiate the wire, do not use force to push the wire.
> - If the wire moves a certain length without any hindrance, then gets stuck—try Wholey wire (Covidien, Mansfield, MA).
> - Do not use Terumo/hydrophilic wire through needle, its Teflon coating will be stripped off.
> - If it does not go after simple maneuvers, remove the needle, press for 10 minutes, then try again either ipsilateral or contralateral side.

Radial Access

Patient Selection

Allen's test: In most of the laboratories, modified Allen's test is used. The steps are:

1. Put a pulse oximeter on the index finger of the right hand—look for normal oximeter wave.

2. Compress the radial artery and look for the response.
   Type A: No change in pulse wave
   Type B: A damped but distinct pulse wave
   Type C: Loss of phasic pulse waveform.

Radial puncture and cannulation can proceed with type A or type B response but not with type C (Fig. 3.9).

Reverse Allen's test: Recommended in previously cannulated radial artery. In this test, phasic waveform is observed after compressing the ulnar artery.

Patient Preparation

Patient to be sedated, well hydrated and comfortably positioned.
- Wrist to be placed next to the femoral access site.
- A roll of sterile towels is used to support and flex the wrist in a hyperextended position (Fig. 3.10).
- *Puncture point:* After draping, radial pulse is palpated. Ideal puncture site is 1–2 cm proximal to radial styloid, the bony prominence of the distal radius.

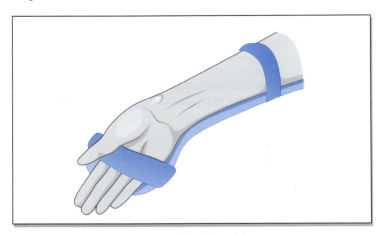

Fig. 3.9: Position of hand for radial puncture

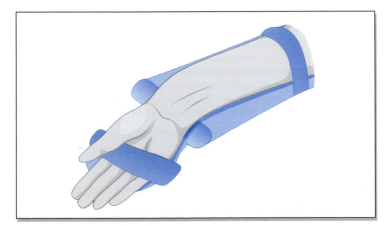

Fig. 3.10: Hyperextension at wrist joint

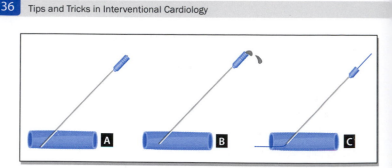

Figs 3.11A to C: Radial artery cannulation

- A small amount (1 mL) of local anesthetic is infiltrated in and around the puncture point, raising a small wheal.
- Many standard radial kits are available nowadays. A standard hydrophilic sheath with Angiocath type 20G needle and 0.25" × 18" cm hydrophilic guidewire (Terumo) can be recommended to start a program.
- The needle with plastic sheath assembly can be steered through the puncture point on the skin towards the artery to transfix the vessel. Once artery is punctured, then there will be a faint blood stain into the needle hub (Fig. 3.11A).
- Remove the needle from the cannula and withdraw the cannula very gently till the pulsatile blood comes out through it (Fig. 3.11B).
- Steer the guidewire through the cannula and keeping guide wire in place, withdraw the cannula from the artery (Fig. 3.11C).
- Make a small nick on the skin around the guidewire with 11-blade scalpel.
- Thread the sheath on the guidewire, till the end of guidewire comes out of the sheath.
- Push the sheath in and remove guidewire and dilator together from the sheath.

Radial Access: Troubleshooting

- If the wire is stuck anywhere, do not push but take an angiogram picture.
- On the basis of angiography, anatomic variant diagnosis is made. This can be classified in three subgroups (Table 3.2):
  1. Group A: Radial-brachial-arterial axis
  2. Group B: Axillary-subclavian-anonymous axis
  3. Group C: Aortic arch
- Commonly a hydrophilic guidewire can overcome tortuosities and bends in Group A. And in Group B, a hydrophilic guidewire and deep inspiration can allow catheter to move into ascending aorta.
- Fact is—Loops and tortuosities are invariably unilateral, so if there is a loop on right side, left radial can be tried.
- Few important tricks can be used before moving to another access:
  1. *Trick 1:* If there is a 360° loop, try with an extra support 0.014 PTCA wire to cross. Try to negotiate with JR catheter, if fails, then—
  2. *Trick 2:* Put another wire to act as a buddy wire and try the same, if fails, then—
  3. *Trick 3:* BAT (Balloon-assisted tracking) is a technique in which an inflated balloon is placed partially into the catheter and partially

Table 3.2: Subgroups of anatomic variant diagnosis

ABC – Anatomical variant	Prevalence
Group A: Radiobrachial arterial axis	
Absent radial pulse	0.3
Significant (>50%) radial stenosis	0.4
Radial-brachial tortuosities (>45°)	4.9
Radial-brachial-arterial loops (Fig. 3.12) (360° loops in arterial course not located at anastomotic sites)	0.4
Radioulnar loops (360° loops at the anastomosis with brachial-ulnar artery)	0.7
High origin of the radial artery, brachial–axillary artery	29
Group B: Axillary subclavian anonymous arterial axis	
Severe tortuosities (bend of >90° in the contour of the vessel)	1.5
Significant (>50%) stenosis	0.4
Group C: Aortic arch	
Retroesophageal right subclavian artery (arteria lusoria)	0.2
Aortic arch elongation	0.1

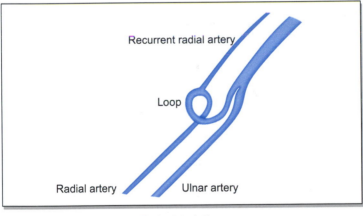

Fig. 3.12: Radial loop

outside, deployed at 3-6 atmosphere pressure. For 5F catheter 1.5 × 15 mm and 6F catheter 2 × 15 mm balloon is used usually. Now entire assembly can be tracked over a 0.014″ PTCA wire. It can be used not only in radial loop but also any spasm or tortuosity involving RA/brachial or subclavian artery.

4. *Trick 4:* Exchange of wire—if it is difficult to track on the PTCA wire—take a pigtail catheter and push the catheter as far as possible, then try to exchange PTCA wire with either 0.025/0.035 wire and try to track on it. Sometimes, the wire can be exchanged with Super Stiff wire and that will straighten the loop. Remember Super Stiff wires precipitate radial spasm (Fig. 3.13).

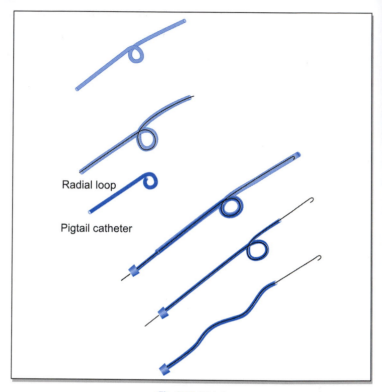

Fig. 3.13: Trick 4

Elongated aorta and arteria lusoria :
True arteria lusoria is rare (<1%) but elongated aorta also, sometimes, has the same effect on transradial procedure. The problems are two-fold:
- To enter ascending aorta
- To cannulate coronary ostium

Entry into ascending aorta (LAO-40 view) (Fig. 3.14):
Ask the patient to take a deep breath, and push the guidewire (0.35). If it enters ascending aorta, track the catheter on it.

    If a right coronary or Tiger cath fail to enter the ascending aorta, take a LIMA diagnostic catheter/Simmons catheter and come to descending aorta. Then rotate the catheter and withdraw so that it faces towards the ascending aorta in LAO view. Push the guidewire and enter ascending aorta. Follow the wire with the catheter. Once in ascending aorta, the catheter is exchanged on an exchange length guidewire (Patel et al.).

Cannulation of coronary arteries:
- *LCA:*
    - EBU, XB (0.5 size larger)
    - JL
    - IKARI L (one size higher)
- *RCA:*
    - MAC, AL, JR.

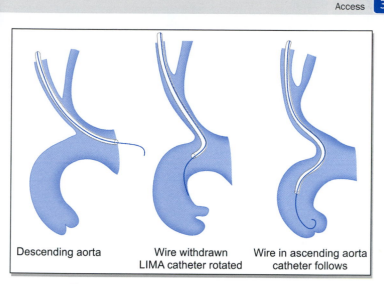

| Descending aorta | Wire withdrawn LIMA catheter rotated | Wire in ascending aorta catheter follows |

Fig. 3.14: Entering ascending aorta from right radial route

Radial Cocktail and Radial Spasm

Radial spasm can make the procedure very uncomfortable both for the patient and the operator. Following are the steps to prevent radial spasm:

1. *Before procedure:*
   a. Topical NTG over the radial artery (optional)
   b. Sedation: Fentanyl – 25–50 µg + Ondansetron 4 mg IV for sedation
   c. Local anesthetic 1% lidocaine
2. *After sheath insertion:*
   a. NTG—100–200 µg/Nicorandil
   b. Verapamil 2.5–5 mg diluted in 10 mL saline
   c. Heparin 5000 IU for angiography and 80–100 IU/kg for PCI
3. • Try to puncture on first attempt
   • Do not exchange catheter frequently
   • Downsizing of catheter (e.g. 5F).

Suggested Reading

1. Francisco Burzotta, et al. Impact of radial-aorta vascular anatomical variants on risk of failure in transradial coronary procedures: Catheter and cardiovascular intervention. 2012;80:298-303.
2. Morton J Kern, et al. Interventional Cardiac Catheterization Handbook: Elsevier. 2013.
3. Patel T, Pancholi S. Working through complexities of radial and brachial vasculature during transradial approach. Catheter and Cardiovascular Intervention (doi:10-1002/ccd 25210).
4. Percutaneous Interventional Cardiovascular Medicine: PCR-EAPCI Textbook, 2012.
5. Tugrul Norgaz, et al. A randomized study comparing effectiveness of right and left radial approach of coronary angiography. Catheter Cardiovascular Intervention. 2012;80:260-64.

Hemodynamics in Cathlab
(The Guiding Star)

■ Shuvanan Ray

Introduction

Hemodynamics is all about pressure, flow, and resistance, the basic factors which governs the function of a simple hydraulic pump—the heart. The pump function is governed by simple law of physics called Darcy's law. The law was formulated by Henry Darcy based on the results of experiments on the flow of water through beds of sand. Darcy's law is a simple mathematical statement, which neatly summarizes the following:

- If there is no pressure gradient over a distance, there is no flow.
- If there is a pressure gradient, flow will occur from high pressure towards low pressure.
- Resistance is the difference in the pressure needed to drive one unit of flow in steady state (mm Hg/mL/min).

$$R = \frac{P_1 - P_2}{Q}$$

The heart as a pump has two basic functions:
1. To pump blood in equal amounts in two systems simultaneously. One is a high pressure and another is a low pressure system.
2. To receive blood simultaneously from two systems, one is oxygenated and another is deoxygenated, both of equal amounts.

How you Formulate Hemodynamic Worksheet?

These are based on calculations derived from data collected through right heart, and sometimes left heart catheterization. The data comprises of:
- Pressure
- Oxygen saturation and content at different points of the heart and the circulation.

From these calculations, the clinician should be able to answer the following questions:
- Is the pump functioning normally?
  1. Receiving normally?
  2. Pumping normally?
  3. Pumping in duress (resistance)?
- Any discrepancy between two sides?

So, hemodynamic principles can be obtained through:
- Pressure measurement by right and left heart catheterization.
- *Cardiac output measurement:*
  - Fick-oxygen method, arterial-venous oxygen difference
  - Indicator—dilution method
  - Indocyanine green
  - Thermodilution.
- Vascular resistance
- Shunt detection and measurement
- Gradients and valve stenosis.

The pressure: Pressure measurements reflect the complex periodic fluctuations in force per unit area, and is measured by fluid-filled catheter manometer. The waveforms are the sum of the forward flow as well as the flow reversal (reflected waves) from the periphery (Fig. 4.1).

Pressure measurement by right heart catheter (Fig. 4.2):
- *Wedge pressure:* Pressure obtained when an end-hole catheter is positioned in a designated vessel with its open end hole facing a capillary bed with no connecting vessels conducting flow into or away from the designated blood vessel between catheter's tip and capillary bed. True wedge pressure can be measured in absence of flow, allowing pressure to equilibrate across capillary bed.
- Catheter can be pulled from the wedge position to PA, RV, RA to measure pressure.
- Simultaneous pressure recording from LV should be taken and following axioms can be obtained from these measurements:

Axioms Derived from Pressure Tracing
- Systolic interval is Q-T and diastolic interval is T-Q.
- Systolic pressure equalization between ventricle and outflow
- Diastolic pressure equalization between atrium and ventricle.
- If there is a pressure drop where equalization is expected—suspect valvular stenosis.
- If there is rise of pressure without pressure drop – suspect regurgitation.
- In absence of tricuspid valve disease, CVP = RA = RVEDP
- In absence of mitral valve disease, PCWP = LA = LVEDP.
  [Actually PCWP is not a very accurate approximation, PCWP < LVEDP {Aortic regurgitation and diastolic dysfunction of LV, when mitral Valve closes prematurely} PCWP> LVEDP {in pulmonary disease, when small vessels constrict due to hypoxia}].

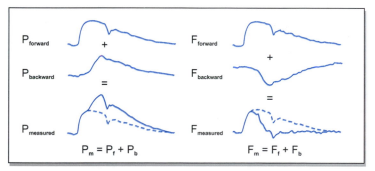

$$P_m = P_f + P_b \qquad F_m = F_f + F_b$$

Fig. 4.1: Central aortic pressure (P) and flow (F) measured during cardiac catheterization

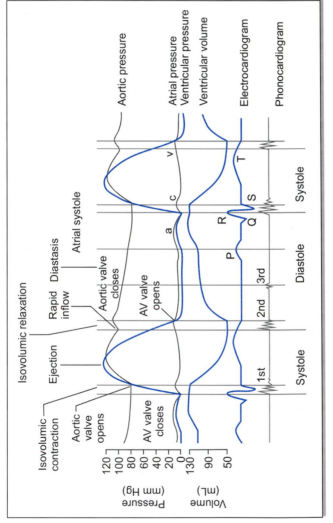

Fig. 4.2: Pressure and volume changes during cardiac cycle with ECG and phonocardiogram

Measurement of Cardiac Output

Cardiac output (CO) is the amount of blood pumped into the outflow of the heart each minute. This is also the quantity of the blood that flow through the circulation each minute. The cardiac output can be measured by Fick's principle (Fig. 4.3).

Thermodilution based on an Indicator–Dilution Methodology (a derivation of Fick's Principle)

Fick's principle is the gold standard for the cardiac output determination and in which cardiac output is O_2 consumption divided by arteriovenous O_2 difference. Although oxygen consumption can be measured quite accurately, the measurement is cumbersome and many laboratories use standard tables for an assumed value instead of direct measurement. Such an estimation may cause an error. Thermodilution is accurate in patients with normal or high output state, but becomes inaccurate in patients with intracardiac shunts, low cardiac output states, significant tricuspid regurgitation or irregular rhythms.

Fick's principle: Fick's principle is explained by Figure 4.3. This figure shows that 200 mL of O_2 are being absorbed from lungs into pulmonary blood each minute. It also shows that O_2 contents of blood entering lungs is 160 mL/L whereas O_2 content of blood leaving the lungs is 200 mL/L. So each liter of blood absorbs 40 mL of O_2 from lungs. Now if, 200 mL of O_2 is absorbed in 1 minute, then 200/40 = 5 L of blood must pass through the lungs each minute, this is the cardiac output.

$$CO = \frac{O_2 \text{ Consumption (VO}_2)}{AV\ O_2 \text{ difference}}$$

So, the easy calculation is:

$VO_2 = 125 \times BSA$ Boys $VO_2 = 138.1 - 1.49 \ln(\text{age}) + 0.378 (HR)$

Girls $VO_2 = 138.1 - 17.04 \ln(\text{age}) + 0.378 (HR)$

$CaO_2 = (1.36 \times Hb\% \times SaO_2)$
$CvO_2 = (1.36 \times Hb\% \times SvO_2)$

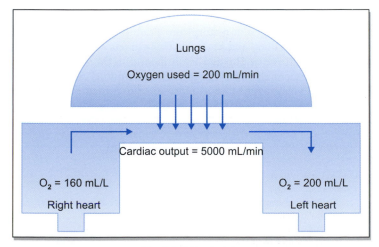

Fig. 4.3: Fick's principle

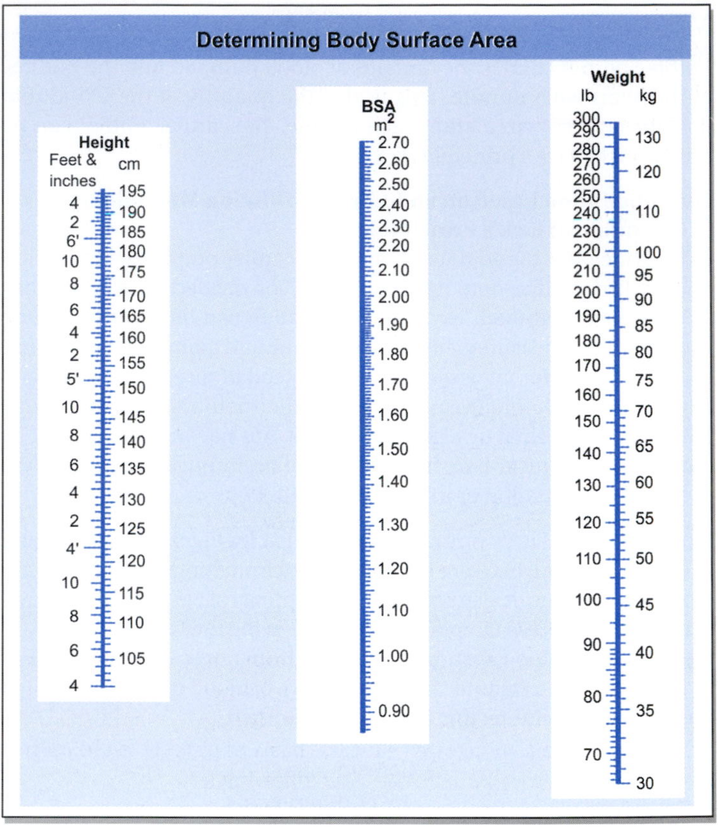

Fig. 4.4: Nomogram

And, $$CO = \frac{(VO_2)}{(CaO_2 - CvO_2) \times 10}$$

BSA can be calculated from height, weight and BSA nomogram (Fig. 4.4)

$$BSA = \sqrt{\{Height\ (cm) \times Weight\ (kg)/3600\}}$$

Assessment of oxygen consumption: Traditionally, this has been measured using a hood and gas pump that extracts all exhaled air and passes it through a mixing system before measuring the oxygen content. This measurement also involves several assumptions (Table 4.1). So for practical work, oxygen consumption is not measured routinely, it is calculated using nomograms as *assumed oxygen consumption* (Table 4.1).

Example:
- 56 years old man
- Height = 180 cm
- Weight = 70 kg
- Oxygen consumption = 250 mL/minute
- Arterial oxygen saturation = 98%
- Venous oxygen saturation = 70%
- Hemoglobin = 14 gm/dL.

Table 4.1: Oximetry run

Site	Average	Range
Superior vena cava (SVC)	74%	67–83%
Inferior vena cava (IVC)	78%	65–87%
Right atrium (RA)	75%	65–87%
Right ventricle (RV)	75%	67–84%
Pulmonary artery (PA)	75%	67–84%
Left atrium (LA)	95%	92–98%
Left ventricle (LV)	95%	92–98%
Femoral artery (FA)	95%	92–98%

Cardiac output = (Oxygen consumption)/(Arterial – Venous O_2 saturation) × 1.36 × Hb% × 10

= 250/(0.98 – 0.70)(1.36)(14)(10)

= 4.69 L/min

BSA = [(Height (cm) × Weight (kg)]/3600)$^{1/2}$ = 1.87 sqm

C1 (L/min/sqm) = C0/BSA = 4.69/1.87 = 2.51 L/min/sqcm

Uses of Hemodynamic Calculations in Cathlab

Calculation of shunt: Detection, localization and quantification of intracardiac shunts are an integral part of hemodynamic evaluation of patients with congenital heart disease. Though in most cases, an intracardiac shunt is suspected on the basis of clinical evaluation of the patient before catheterization. The following data obtained during catheterization should alert cardiologist to look for a shunt that had not been suspected previously (Tables 4.2 and 4.3).

- Unexplained arterial desaturation (?R–L shunt)
- Unexpectedly high (> 80%) PA saturation (?L–R shunt)

Many different techniques are available for the detection, localization and quantification of left to right intracardiac shunts but measurement of oxygen saturation and content (oximetry run) is the most commonly used method (Table 4.4).

Samples need to be acquired with the patient breathing (or being ventilated with) air or a gas mixture containing no more than a maximum of 30% oxygen. Saturation data will be inaccurate, if oxygen enriched gas (> 30% oxygen) is being given due to significantly increased dissolved oxygen in pulmonary venous sample, which will overestimate the pulmonary flow.

During a routine heart catheterization, two blood samples will be obtained: (1) SVC and (2) pulmonary artery. In absence of LR shunt, the PA saturation represents the best measurement of MVO_2 (mixed venous O_2 saturation). In presence of LR shunt, MVO_2 is the O_2 saturation of the chamber just proximal to the shunt, i.e. proximal to O_2 step up (Table 4.4).

- MVO_2 is < 60 to 65%, it correlates with increased O_2 extraction by tissues as in low cardiac output states, shock states or anemia.

In oximetry run normally O_2 saturation is measured:

PA = RV = RA = Average of SVC and IVC $\dfrac{(3 \times SVC + 1 \times IVC)}{4}$ (Flamm's equation)

SVC O_2 saturation is lower than IVC (Renal tissues extract very less O_2)

Table 4.2: Basic calculations derived from cardiac output

Vascular resistance	Use only mean pressure
PVR = Pulmonary vascular resistance	$\dfrac{PA - PCWP}{CO}$
SVR = Systemic vascular resistance	$\dfrac{AO - RA}{CO}$

PA mean pressure =	$\dfrac{PASP + 2\,PADP}{3}$
Mean arterial pressure =	Diastolic pressure + 1/3 pulse pressure

Table 4.3: Normal hemodynamic values

Flows	
Cardiac Index	2.6–4.2 (L/min/m²)
Stroke volume Index	35–55 mL/m²
Pressure (in mm Hg)	
Aorta (S/D/M)	100–140/60–90/70–105
LV (S/ED)	100–140/3–12
LA (PCWP)	
Mean	1–10
a Wave	3–15
v Wave	3–15
PA (S/D/M)	15–30/2–8/10–15
RV (S/ED)	15–30/2–8
RA	
Mean	2–8
a Wave	2–10
v Wave	2–10
Resistances	
SVR	10–20 (woods unit) or 770–1500 (dynes)
PVR	0.25–1.5 (woods unit) or 20–120 (dynes)
O₂ Consumption	110–150 (mL/min/m²)
AVO₂ Difference	3–4.5 (mL/dL)

Table 4.4: Oximetry run obtain 2 mL sample from each of the following locations

• Left and/or right pulmonary artery
• MPA
• RV outflow tract
• RV mid area
• RV (Tricuspid valve or apex)
• RA—Low (near TV) + Mid + High
• SVC—Low (near RA junction) + High (near junction of in nominate vein)
• IVC—High (just at or below diaphragm)
• IVC—Low (at L_{4-5})
• LV
• Aorta (distal to insertion of ductus)

Oxygen saturation step-up: > 8% between SVC and PA is indicative of a significant shunt. Once a shunt is detected a full oximetry run should be performed.

Oxygen Saturation Abnormalities

• Elevated PA saturation	• High cardiac output • LR shunt
• Low PA saturation	• Low cardiac output • Low systemic arterial saturation • Increased oxygen extraction
• Elevated FA saturation	• Patient-receiving oxygen
• Low FA saturation	• Lung disease • Pulmonary edema • RL shunt

Left to Right Shunt Oximetry Run (Table 4.5)

Normally, PVO_2 is equal to SAO_2 (arterial saturation), if there is no bidirectional or RL shunt. The presence of such shunts will be suspected when SAO_2 is lower than PVO_2 (in the later cases, PVO_2 may be considered 98% in absence of lung disease or pulmonary edema). In patients with arterial saturation < 95% in absence of lung diseases or hypoventilation should be evaluated for presence of bidirectional or RL shunt.

The most important calculations for practical purpose is probably the pulmonary to systemic flow ratio (Qp/Qs). This provides simple and reliable estimate of the extent to which the pulmonary flow is increased or reduced.

$$Qp : Qs = \frac{Sat\ A_O - Sat\ MV}{Sat\ PV - Sat\ PA}$$

Beyond infancy, if $Qp/Qs \geq 1.8 : 1$ in a shunt, it requires intervention. While one of $\leq 1.5 : 1$ may be regarded as insignificant. A flow ratio < 1 indicates RL shunt and is often a sign of irreversible pulmonary vascular disease.

Table 4.5: L-R Shunt—oximetry run

Level of shunt	Mean of distal chamber samples (O_2 saturation %)	Possible causes of step up
Atrial (SVC/IVC to RA)	≥7	ASD, partial anomalous pulmonary venous drainage, RSOV, VSD with TR, coronary fistula to RA
Ventricular (RA to RV)	≥5	VSD, PDA with PR, ostium primum ASD, coronary fistula to RV
Great vessels (RV to PA)	≥5	PDA, AP window, aberrant coronary artery origin
Any level (SVC to PA)	≥7	All of the above

Unexplained arterial desaturation should immediately raise the suspicion of a right to left intracardiac shunt. Most commonly arterial desaturations (O_2 sat < 95%) detected during cardiac catheterization represents alveolar ventilation (associated with excessive sedation, pulmonary parenchymal disease or pulmonary congestion or edema secondary to the patient's cardiac disease. These problems are exacerbated by supine position and helping the patient to assume a more upright posture, encouraging the patient to take deep breaths and to cough will correct or substantially ameliorate arterial hypoxemia in most cases. If arterial desaturation persists, oxygen should be administered by facemask—especially non re-breathing mask). If full arterial blood saturation cannot be achieved by facemask administration RL shunt is presumed to be present.

Bidirectional shunt: Once a shunt is diagnosed with a Qp : Qs ratio < 1, it signifies a net right to left shunt, but a Qp : Qs ratio $\leq$ 1.5 may not always signify a small shunt, it may be a significant bidirectional shunting.

Suspicion of Right to Left Shunt (Flow chart 4.1)

Flow chart 4.1: Suspicion of RL shunt

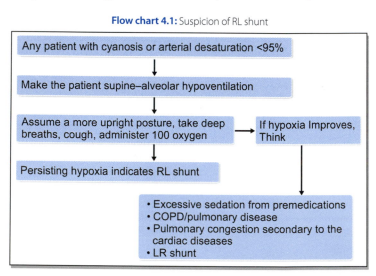

Right to Left Shunt Oximetry

- The site of RL shunt may be localized, if blood samples can be obtained from pulmonary valve, LA, LV and aorta
- Pulmonary valve blood of patients with RL shunt is fully saturated with oxygen
- The site of a RL shunt may be localized by noting which left heart chamber first to show desaturation (step down)
- Qeff Calculation quantifies RL shunt (Qs – Qeff)

Calculation of RL and Bidirectional Shunt

If there is evidence of a RL shunt, as well as LR shunt, a quick approximation can be obtained by using a hypothetic quantity known as effective blood flow, the flow that would exist in the absence of any shunt.

Table 4.6: Calculation of Qeff (effective pulmonary flow)

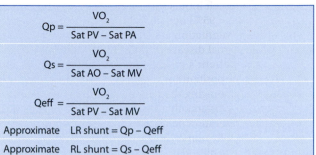

$$Qp = \dfrac{VO_2}{Sat\ PV - Sat\ PA}$$	
$$Qs = \dfrac{VO_2}{Sat\ AO - Sat\ MV}$$	
$$Qeff = \dfrac{VO_2}{Sat\ PV - Sat\ MV}$$	
Approximate	LR shunt = Qp – Qeff
Approximate	RL shunt = Qs – Qeff

Q_{eff} (Effective Pulmonary Flow) (Table 4.6)

If there is a significant LR shunt (more than RL shunt) in a case with bidirectional shunting, pulmonary and systemic vascular resistance should be calculated.

Next very important calculation is determination of resistance:
If PVR is > 6 woods unit or > 2/3rd of SVR, pulmonary vaso-reactivity testing is indicated to rule out Eisenmenger syndrome. If with 100% oxygen inhalation, mean PA pressure decreases > 10 mm Hg or comes below 40 mm Hg. and PVR reduces > 20% or comes below 5 woods unit—the shunt should be closed.

Calculation of Valve Areas

Normally, the LA pressure and LV end-diastolic pressure equalizes in diastole. The normal mitral valve area is 3–4 cm², but when it is reduced to < 2 cm², the LA–LV gradient is established and when it is <1 cm² there appears a significant pressure gradient at rest and pulmonary hypertension develops.

Similarly, normal aortic valve is 3–4 cm², if the valve area is < 1 cm², then symptoms of aortic stenosis develops.

Tricuspid valve area is 7 cm², if it is < 1.5 cm², gradient appears. And when it is < 1 cm² and mean RA pressure > 10 mm Hg—patient develops peripheral edema.

In pulmonary valve, peak-to-peak pressure difference is measured.
If the gradient is < 50 mm Hg   = Mild pulmonary stenosis
                                50–100 mm Hg = Moderate pulmonary stenosis
                                > 100 mm Hg   = Severe pulmonary stenosis

The valve orifice area can often be estimated by a formula developed by Dr Richards Gorlin. If the mean pressure gradient, the cardiac output and the systolic ejection period (from semilunar opening to closure)/diastolic filling period (AV valve opening to closure) are known, and if the patient is not in low cardiac output state:

$$\text{Valve orifice area (cm}^2) = \frac{\text{Cardiac output}}{(\text{SFP/DFP}) \times HR \times 44.3/37.7 \times \sqrt{(\text{mean gradient})}}$$

SEP/DFP is calculated by measuring at 100 mm/sec paper speed.

Empiric constant in formula for 2 leaflets is 37.7 and for 3 leaflets is 44.3.

Gorlin formula is cumbersome. So for practical purposes, Hakki formula is substituted.

$$\text{Hakki valve orifice area (cm}^2) = \frac{\text{Cardiac output (L/min)}}{\sqrt{\text{(Pressure gradient)}}}$$

The Angel correction mandates that above result be divided by 1.35 for a HR< 75/min or >90/min in setting of aortic stenosis.

- *For aortic stenosis:* Hakki formula involves peak-to-peak gradient and for mitral valve area involves mean pressure gradient.

Multiple pressure measurements—classic signs of disease processes
- Constrictive pericarditis veruss restrictive cardiomyopathy (Table 4.7)
- Aortic regurgitation (Fig. 4.5)
- Mitral regurgitation (Fig. 4.6)
- Carabello's sign (Severe AS) (Fig. 4.7)
- Brockenbrough sign (Fig. 4.8)
- Wide pulse pressure (aortic systolic pressure—diastolic pressure > 70 mm Hg) is classical for aortic regurgitation (Fig. 4.5).
- Early large 'v' wave bisecting down stroke of LV—Classical for MR (Fig. 4.6)
- Increase in aortic pressure after withdrawal of catheter from LV: Carabello's sign, classical for severe AS (Fig. 4.7)
- Brockenbrough-Braunwald-Morrow sign (Fig. 4.8)

The peak systolic gradient rise after an ectopic beat in simultaneous pressure tracing of aorta and LV but with decrease in pulse pressure—classical for HOCM.

Table 4.7: Hemodynamic differentiation of restrictive cardiomyopathy versus constrictive pericarditis

	Constrictive pericarditis	Restricitve cardiomyopathy
EDP equalization (LVEDP-RVEDP)	< 5 mm Hg	> 5 mm Hg
PA pressure	< 55 mm Hg	> 55 mm Hg
RVEDP/RVSP	> 1/3	< 1/3
Dip-Plateau morphology (square root sign)	LV rapid filling wave > 7 mm Hg	LV rapid filling wave < 7 mm Hg
Respiratory variation	No respiratory variation in mean RAP	Normal respiratory variation in mean RAP

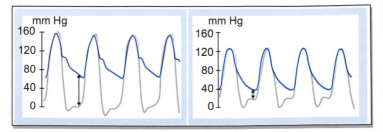

Fig. 4.5: Simultaneous aortic and LV pressure measurement in normal and in AR

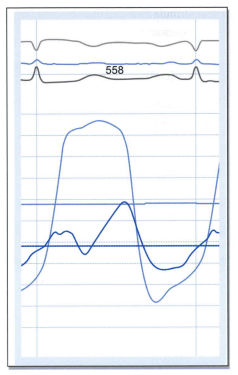

Fig. 4.6: Large V wave in mitral regurgitation

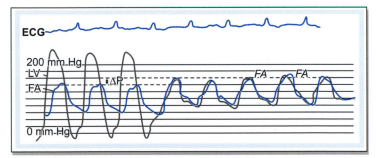

Fig. 4.7: Carabello's sign in aortic stenosis

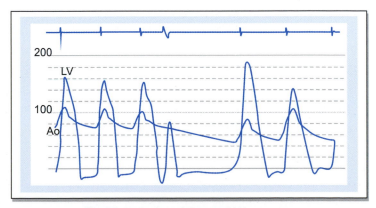

Fig. 4.8: Brockenbrough-Braunwald-Morrow sign

Suggested Reading

1. Akram M, Ajmi A. Invasive hemodynamic manual for adult cardiac catheterization, 2013.
2. Grossman and Baim's Cardiac catheterization and angiography. Mauro Moscucci; Lippincott & Wilkins, 8th Edition, 2014.
3. Textbook of Medical Physiology. Guyton and Hall, 11th edn. Sounders, 2006.

Vascular Anatomy and Radiographic Views (The Pathway)

■ Sabyasachi Mitra, Shuvanan Ray

Heart

The heart is a hollow muscular organ that is somewhat pyramid shaped and lies within the pericardium in the mediastinum. It is connected at its base to the great blood vessels but otherwise lies free within the pericardium.

Chambers of the Heart

The heart is divided by vertical septa into four chambers: the right and left atria and the right and left ventricles. The right atrium lies anterior to the left atrium, and the right ventricle lies anterior to the left ventricle.

The walls of the heart are composed of cardiac muscle—the *myocardium* covered externally with serous pericardium; the *epicardium* and lined internally with a layer of endothelium; and the *endocardium*.

Right Atrium

The right atrium consists of a main cavity and a small outpouching, the auricle.

Openings into the right atrium: The *superior vena cava* and the *inferior vena cava* (larger than the superior vena cava) opens into the upper and lower part of the right atrium; and returns the blood to the heart from the upper and lower half of the body, respectively. The *coronary sinus*, which drains most of the blood from the heart wall, opens into the right atrium between the inferior vena cava and the atrioventricular orifice. The *right atrioventricular orifice* lies anterior to the inferior vena caval opening and is guarded by the tricuspid valve. Many small orifices of small veins also drain the wall of the heart and open directly into the right atrium.

Right Ventricle

The right ventricle communicates with the right atrium through the atrioventricular orifice and with the pulmonary trunk through the pulmonary orifice.

The *tricuspid valve* guards the atrioventricular orifice and consists of three cusps formed by a fold of endocardium with some connective tissue enclosed: *anterior, septal,* and *inferior* (posterior) cusps.

The *pulmonary valve* guards the pulmonary orifice and consists of three semilunar cusps formed by folds of endocardium with some connective tissue enclosed.

Left Atrium

Similar to the right atrium, the left atrium consists of a main cavity and a left auricle. The left atrium is situated behind the right atrium and forms the greater part of the base or the posterior surface of the heart.

Openings into the left atrium: The four pulmonary veins, two from each lung, open through the posterior wall and have no valves.

The left atrioventricular orifice is guarded by the mitral valve.

Left Ventricle

The left ventricle communicates with the left atrium through the atrioventricular orifice and with the aorta through the aortic orifice. The walls of the left ventricle are three times thicker than those of the right ventricle (the left intraventricular blood pressure is six times higher than that inside the right ventricle).

The *mitral valve* guards the atrioventricular orifice. It consists of two cusps, one anterior and one posterior.

The *aortic valve* guards the aortic orifice and is precisely similar in structure to the pulmonary valve. One cusp is situated on the anterior wall (right cusp) and two are located on the posterior wall (left and posterior cusps). Behind each cusp, the aortic wall bulges to form an *aortic sinus*. The anterior aortic sinus gives origin to the right coronary artery, and the left posterior sinus gives origin to the left coronary artery.

Arterial Supply of the Heart

The arterial supply of the heart is provided by the right and left coronary arteries, which arise from the ascending aorta immediately above the aortic valve. The arteries as indicated by their name, form an oblique inverted crown, with an anastomotic circle in the atrioventricular sulcus, connected by marginal and interventricular loops, intersecting at the cardiac apex. The coronary arteries and their major branches are distributed over the surface of the heart, lying within subepicardial connective tissue.

Right Coronary Artery

The *right coronary artery* arises from the anterior aortic sinus of the ascending aorta and runs forward between the pulmonary trunk and the right auricle. It descends almost vertically in the right atrioventricular groove, and at the inferior border of the heart it continues posteriorly along the atrioventricular groove to anastomose with the left coronary artery in the posterior interventricular groove. The following branches from the right coronary artery supply the right atrium and right ventricle and parts of the left atrium and left ventricle and the atrioventricular septum.

Branches

- The *right conus artery* supplies the anterior surface of the pulmonary conus (infundibulum of the right ventricle) and the upper part of the anterior wall of the right ventricle.

- The *anterior ventricular branches* are two or three in number and supply the anterior surface of the right ventricle.

  The *marginal branch* is the largest and runs along the lower margin of the costal surface to reach the apex.
- The *posterior ventricular branches* are usually two in number and supply the diaphragmatic surface of the right ventricle.
- The *posterior interventricular (descending) artery* runs toward the apex in the posterior interventricular groove. It gives off branches to the right and left ventricles, including its inferior wall. It supplies branches to the posterior part of the ventricular septum but not to the apical part, which receives its supply from the anterior interventricular branch of the left coronary artery.

  A large septal branch supplies the *atrioventricular node*. In 10% of individuals, the posterior interventricular artery is replaced by a branch from the left coronary artery.
- The *atrial branches* supply the anterior and lateral surfaces of the right atrium. One branch supplies the posterior surface of both the right and left atria. The *artery of the sinoatrial node* supplies the node and the right and left atria; in 35% of individuals it arises from the left coronary artery.

Left Coronary Artery

The *left coronary artery*, which is usually larger than the right coronary artery, supplies the major part of the heart, including the greater part of the left atrium, left ventricle, and ventricular septum. It arises from the left posterior aortic sinus of the ascending aorta and passes forward between the pulmonary trunk and the left auricle. It then enters the atrioventricular groove and divides into an *anterior interventricular branch and a circumflex branch*.

Branches

- The *anterior interventricular (descending) branch or left anterior descending branch* runs downward in the anterior interventricular groove to the apex of the heart. In most individuals, it then passes around the apex of the heart to enter the posterior interventricular groove and anastomoses with the terminal branches of the right coronary artery. In one-third of individuals, it ends at the apex of the heart. The anterior interventricular branch supplies the right and left ventricles with numerous branches that also supply the anterior part of the ventricular septum. One of these ventricular branches *(left diagonal artery)* may arise directly from the trunk of the left coronary artery. A small *left conus artery* supplies the pulmonary conus.
- The *circumflex artery* is the same size as the left-anterior descending artery. It winds around the left margin of the heart in the atrioventricular groove. A *left marginal artery* is a large branch that supplies the left margin of the left ventricle down to the apex. *Anterior ventricular* and *posterior ventricular branches* supply the left ventricle. *Atrial branches* supply the left atrium. In *left dominance*, the posterior interventricular artery is a branch of the circumflex branch of the left coronary artery (10%) (see right coronary artery).

Anomalous Coronary Arteries during Angiography

Origin of both coronary arteries from same sinus of Valsalva.

The anomalous artery has either of the four types (Fig. 5.1):

1. *Type A:* Anterior to pulmonary trunk.
2. *Type B:* Between aorta and pulmonary trunk.
3. *Type C:* Through crista supraventricularis (within ventricular septum).
4. *Type D:* Dorsal to the aorta.
   Angiographic appearance is shown in Figure 5.1.
   Type B and type C vessels are prone to ischemia due to shape of the coronary ostium of the anomalous vessel which is slit-like instead of normal round shape. Clinical events, including even sudden death occur during exercise, particularly in young adults.

Purpose of Angiography before PCI is to Delineate

- Selection of appropriate guide catheter.
- Target vessels, pathway and angle of entry.
- Lesion length and morphology using additional angulated views eliminating vessel overlap.
- Degree of ostial atherosclerosis.
- Assessment of collaterals.
- True (maximally vasodilated) diameter of the target vessel.

There are few general rules for radiographic visualization

- Left circumflex artery (LCX) goes with image intensifier [in left anterior oblique (LAO) view LCX is left side of screen and vice versa, similarly caudal view LCX is below and vice versa).
- Left anterior descending (LAD) goes opposite to image intensifier (in LAO view, LAD is on the right side of screen).
- Spine and diaphragm moves with image intensifier (LAO—they are on the left side of screen).

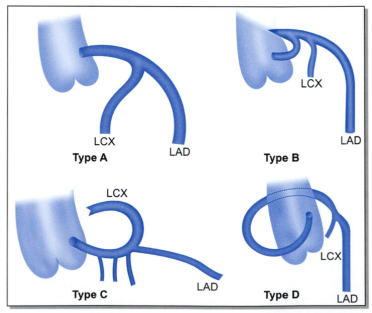

Fig. 5.1: Types of anomalous coronary arteries

How to Start Coronary Visualization?

To start with it is better to have a neutral view like AP which gives an idea about LM (its ostium, shaft, bifurcation) and its branches, particularly the LCX.

Now from AP (Fig. 5.2):

- *If the LCX is lower than LAD:* Best view to expose LCX is AP caudal or shallow LAO (10–15°) caudal and with deep inspiration. This will expose LCX without much foreshortening.
- *If the LCX is above LAD:* Still for LCX mid and distal part, it is better to have AP caudal or RAO caudal views in deep inspiration. For proximal LAD or LCX, LAO caudal (Spider) will be an essential view. It will show both the ostia (LAD/LCX), helps to wire both the branches of left main coronary artery (LMCA), proximal branches of LAD (D1) or LCX (OM1).
- *Views to expose LAD:* 2 views that expose the LAD, particularly, the mid and distal parts are:
    1. AP cranial/shallow RAO cranial views
    2. LAO cranial views (Fig. 5.3).

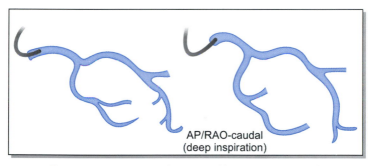

Fig. 5.2: Anteroposterior/right anterior oblique (AP/RAO)—caudal

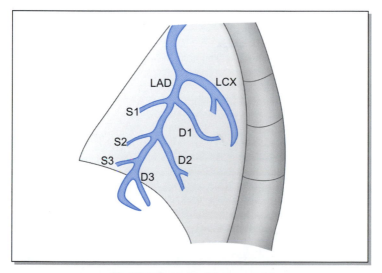

Fig. 5.3: Left anterior oblique—cranial

The proximal LAD is usually foreshortened in LAO cranial views, but AP/RAO cranial views expose the artery nicely. The LAO cranial is also very important to visualize the septal and diagonal separation; but it needs a little manipulation to have the best picture. The artery appears to be straight in this view and the LAO and cranial both should be manipulated with patient taking deep inspiration in such a way that the artery is placed in the translucent triangle bound by spine on the left and diaphragm right and down and edge of the intensifier above.

Proximal LAD: If in AP view LCX is lower than LAD then RAO/AP caudal views expose the proximal LAD fully, but if there are multiple overlaps on LAD in AP view then either AP cranial with deep inspiration (moves LCX above) or LAO cranial (Spider) views expose proximal LAD. Sometimes, a deep RAO and deep cranial (above 40° each) can expose LAD from ostium to tip with all its branches (Fig. 5.4, Table 5.1).

Right coronary artery (RCA): In routine angiography usually a LAO 30° can give an overall assessment of the artery. LAO cranial view can show the distal bifurcation whereas the LAO caudal view can show the ostial and proximal part better (Fig. 5.5, Table 5.2).

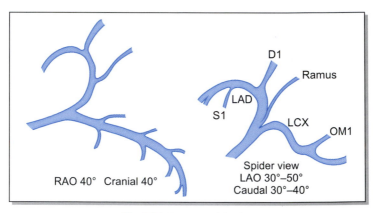

Fig. 5.4: Left coronary injection

Table 5.1: Summary of angiographic views of left coronary artery

		Routine	*Back-up*
LMCA	Ostium	AP/AP caudal	LAO RAO 10° steep cranial
	Body	RAO 30°, cranial 20° LAO 15° steep cranial	AP caudal RAO 30°, caudal 20°
	Distal	LAO 30–50° caudal 30°/40° (Spider)	
LAD	Ostial	Spider view	RAO 40°, cranial 40°
	Proximal	LAO 15° steep cranial RAO 15° shallow caudal	AP caudal
	Mid and Distal	AP cranial 30°	RAO 20°/30° Cranial 30°/40°
LCX	Ostium	Spider view	RAO 30° shallow caudal
	Body	RAO 20° shallow caudal AP caudal 30°	LAO 10° steep caudal

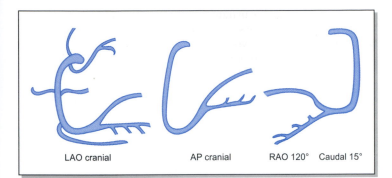

Fig. 5.5: Right coronary artery injection

Table 5.2: Summary of angiographic views for RCA

	Routine	*Back-up*
Proximal	LAO	RAO
	LAO caudal	AP caudal
Mid	LAO	Lateral
	RAO	
Distal	LAO cranial	AP cranial
	AP cranial	Deep RAO shallow caudal

RAO view (30–40°) shows proximal and mid-segment of RCA, and sometimes used to assess the coaxiality of JR catheter in the ostium or separate the branches in the middle from the main RCA.

AP cranial view is occasionally needed to assess the PDA/PLB ostium and body.

Deep RAO with mild caudal (RAO 120° with caudal 15°) sometimes needed to assess distal part better as left lateral occasionally for mid part.

Angiography for Postcoronary Artery Bypass Grafting (CABG) Patients

A vein graft can usually be entered as ostium visualized in LAO 40–70° and RAO 30–40° projections. The principle of selecting the best angle for a venous or arterial graft is to angle a perpendicular view from the direction of the bypass graft. Reverse saphenous vein graft (RSVG) to RCA/LAD is best seen in LAO view while RSVG to OM is best seen in RAO view.

The cranial and caudal angulations are sometimes necessary to visualize part of the graft better which is summarized in Table 5.3.

Coronary Lesions for PCI

The ACC-AHA classified the lesions in 2000 according to the risk in PCI stent era (mainly depending on ability of stent to manage initial or subsequent complications of coronary interventions) summarized below:

Low risk
- Discrete (length < 10 mm)
- Concentric

Table 5.3: Grafts

IMA graft	Ostium	Straight AP
	Body	Straight AP RAO—15° shallow caudal
	Distal anastomosis	Left lateral AP cranial
RCA venous graft	Ostium	LAO 20° shallow cranial
	Body	LAO/RAO (30°)
	Distal	LAO/AP cranial Lateral, RAO cranial
LAD RSVG	Ostium	LAO 45°
	Body	LAO 45° RAO 30° Left lateral
	Distal	Left lateral AP/RAO—15° steep cranial
LCX	Ostium	LAO 45°
	Body	LAO 45°
	Distal	RAO cranial, AP caudal

- Readily accessible
- Nonangulated segment (< 45°)
- Smooth Contour
- Little or no calcification
- Less than totally occlusive
- Not ostial in location
- No major side branch involvement
- Absence of thrombus.

Moderate risk
- Tubular (length 10–20 mm)
- Eccentric
- Moderate tortuosity of proximal segment
- Moderately angulated segment (> 45°, < 90°)
- Irregular contour
- Moderate or heavy calcification
- Total occlusion < 3 months old
- Ostial in location
- Bifurcation lesions requiring double guidewires
- Some thrombus present (Table 5.4).

High risk
- Diffuse (length > 20 mm)
- Excessive tortuosity of proximal segment
- Extremely angulated segments > 90°
- Total occlusions > 3 months old/bridging collaterals
- Inability to protect major side branches
- Degenerated vein grafts with friable lesions (Table 5.4).

A Few Words about Coronary Calcification

Coronary calcification particularly in and around a lesion is very important finding, as it can modify the strategy of PCI. Coronary

Table 5.4: Angiographic calcification (Yoshinobu Onua, 2010)

Severe	Radio-opacities noted without cardiac motion prior to contrast injection, generally involving both sides of arterial wall (rail track calcification)
Moderate	Densities noted only during cardiac cycle prior to contrast injection
Mild	Lesions other than moderate or severe

Table 5.5: The thrombolysis in myocardial infarction (TIMI) thrombus scale

Grade 0	No angiographic evidence of thrombus
Grade 1	Angiographic features suggestive of thrombus
	• Decreased contrast density
	• Haziness of contrast
	• Irregular lesion contour
	• A smooth convex meniscus at the site of total occlusion
	Suggestive, but not firmly diagnostic of thrombus
Grade 2	Definite thrombus present in multiple angiographic projections Marked irregular lesion contour with a significant filling defect—the thrombus Greatest dimension is less than ½ vessel dimension
Grade 3	Definite thrombus appears in multiple views Greatest dimension > ½ to < 2 vessel dimension
Grade 4	Definite large thrombus present Greatest dimension > 2 vessel dimension
Grade 5	Definite complete thrombotic occlusion of a vessel A convex margin that stains with contrast, persisting for several cardiac cycles

calcification is not always picked up by angiography. However, an angiographic calcification assessment was done SPIRIT-II study and the results summarized in Table 5.5.

Angiography is not the ideal tool for detection of coronary thrombus but thrombus detected during angiography has been shown to be associated with adverse procedural outcomes, such as no reflow, distal embolization and abrupt closure. Angiographic thrombus grading is summarized in Table 5.4. In patients with occluded artery, thrombus is reclassified into STB (small thrombus burden) or LTB (large thrombus burden), after flow achievement with guidewire crossing or a small (1.5 mm) deflated balloon passage or dilatation. STB (when thrombus < G4) and LTB (G4) are correlated with clinical outcomes.

Angiographic TIMI Classification of Blood Flow

The PCI is all about restoring the flow across the coronary artery. It is well known that only patency of the artery does not ensure normal flow. To assess the flow, TIMI flow grading (Tables 5.6 and 5.7) has been used which gives a qualitative assessment of the flow through the coronary arteries.

Syntax score: SYNTAX trial compared multivessel PCI with left main narrowing to PCI in 2009. The angiograms of the patients were

Table 5.6: Thrombolysis in myocardial infarction (TIMI)—Flow grade

TIMI flow grade	Description
TIMI-0 (No perfusion)	No antegrade flow beyond occlusion
TIMI-1 (Penetration without perfusion)	Contrast hangs up just beyond the obstruction and fails to opacify the distal coronary bed during the cine run
TIMI-2 (Partial perfusion)	Contrast fills the distal coronary tree but rate of entry/clearance from the distal vessel is slower than comparable arteries not perfused by culprit artery
TIMI-3 (Complete perfusion)	Antegrade flow into the distal artery as promptly as into the bed proximal to the obstruction and clearance from the involved bed is as rapid as from uninvolved bed in the same vessel or the opposite artery

Table 5.7: TIMI—Myocardial perfusion grading (TMPG)

TMPG 0 :	Dye fails to enter the microvasculature of the involved artery (No ground glass opacification)
TMPG 1:	Dye slowly enters but fails to exit. The ground glass opacity remains there as a stain even after disappearance of dye from the vessel
TMPG 2:	Delayed entry/exit of dye from the microvasculature. The ground glass opacification is not cleared within 3 cardiac cycles (does not or minimally diminishes in intensity)
TMPG 3 :	Normal entry/exit of dye. Washout within 3 cardiac cycles or markedly diminished after that

analyzed by a particular scoring system, an angiographic grading tool to determine the complexity of CAD. It was derived from pre-existing lesion classification by ACC-AHA, AHA classification of coronary artery tree segments, total occlusion classification system, Duke and international classification for patient safety (ICPS) classification system for bifurcation lesion and a consensus opinion from among the world experts.

Syntax score is the sum of the points assigned to each individual lesion with > 50% diameter in vessels > 1.5 mm diameter. Coronary tree is divided into 16 segments according to AHA classification. Each segment is given a score to 1 or 2 based on the presence of the disease. A value of five given to LMCA, 3.5 to proximal LAD and 0.5 for smaller branches. Total occlusion > 3 months duration, features for procedural difficulty like blunt stump, bridging collaterals and a side branch > 1.5 mm diameter all gets 1 point. Bifurcation, trifurcation gets additional points depending upon segments involved. Similarly aorto-ostial, vessel tortuosity, length of lesion > 20 mm and calcification all gets additional points, the syntax score algorithm then seems each of these features for a total syntax score and it is available as a computer algorithm on line: According to the trial SYNTAX score < 18 PCI may be even better than coronary artery bypass graft (CABG) with similar major cardiac events with lower stroke rate whereas high SYNTAX score > 34 coronary artery bypass grafting is better compared to PCI.

Angiographic Classification of Collateral Flow

Collaterals can be seen angiographically with late opacification of a totally or sub-totally occluded blood vessel (Fig. 5.6). They may be antegrade or retrograde. Retrograde channels can be used to cross chronic total occlusion (CTO) retrogradely or to place guidewire into the true lumen during antegrade approach. Assessment of collaterals are also important in decision making of PCI. The donor artery should be protected first. Angiographic classification is graded as follows (Table 5.8):

Werner classification of coronary collaterals (Important in retrograde wiring in CTO)

CC–0:   Coronary collateral with no visible connection to the recipient artery

CC–1:   Tiny or faint CC connection

CC–2:   Small vessel like connection

Coronary ectasia/aneurysm: Dilatation of an arterial segment to a diameter at least 1.5 times that of adjacent normal coronary artery, it can be either diffuse affecting the entire length of a coronary artery or localized. It is attributed to atherosclerosis in 50% of cases, whereas

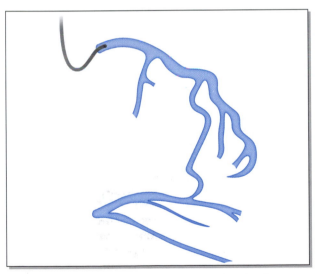

Fig. 5.6: In RAO cranial view, the classic septal coronary collateral (CC) connecting LAD and PDA has a classic 'b-shape' distal turn near its connection. This course should be looked for when advancing the wire

Table 5.8: Coronary collaterals—Angiographic classification (Rentrop)

Grade 0	No collateral branches seen
Grade 1	Very weak (ghost-like) opacification is seen
Grade 2	Opacified segment is less dense than donor vessel and filling slowly
Grade 3	Opacified segment is as dense as the donor vessel and filling rapidly

20–30% are considered to be congenital in origin. In the great majority of these patients ectasia co-exists with CAD. Only 10–20% of CAE have been decided in association with inflammation or coronary artery disease.

Pulmonary Trunk

Branches

The pulmonary trunk conveys deoxygenated blood, from the right ventricle to the lungs. It divides into the right and left pulmonary arteries, of almost equal size. The right part slightly longer and larger, reaches the right pulmonary hilum, where it bifurcates. The lower larger branch is distributed to the middle and lower lobes, while the upper branch accompanies the right upper lobar bronchus. The left pulmonary artery, shorter and smaller, runs horizontally, dividing into upper and lower lobar branches at the hilum.

Arch of the Aorta

The arch of the aorta is a continuation of the ascending aorta. It lies behind the manubrium sterni and arches upward, backward, and to the left in front of the trachea (its main direction is backward). It then passes downward to the left of the trachea and, at the level of the sternal angle, becomes continuous with the descending aorta.

Branches

The *brachiocephalic artery* arises from the convex surface of the aortic arch. It passes upward and to the right of the trachea and divides into the right subclavian and right common carotid arteries behind the right sternoclavicular joint. The *left common carotid artery* arises from the convex surface of the aortic arch on the left side of the brachiocephalic artery. It runs upward and to the left of the trachea and enters the neck behind the left sternoclavicular joint. The *left subclavian artery* arises from the aortic arch behind the left common carotid artery. It runs upward along the left side of the trachea and the esophagus to enter the root of the neck. It arches over the apex of the left lung.

Radiological Appearance

The shadow of the arch is easily identified in AP view and the left profile is called the aortic knuckle.

Assessment of aortic arch anatomy is crucial. With increasing age, the aorta tends to unfold and elongate, with great vessels origin being displaced caudally. This creates a steeper aortic arch over time and spreads the origins of great vessels as well as altering their angle of take off, relative to the top of the arch. The aortic arch is classified into 3 categories: Type I, II and III, based on the degree of inferior displacement of the great vessels from the top curvature of the arch. Type I aortic arch is where all three great vessels are originating in the same horizontal planes. In type II, the innominate artery originates between the horizontal planes of the outer and inner curvatures of the aortic arch. In Type III, the innominate artery originates below the horizontal plane of inner curvature of aortic arch (Fig. 5.7).

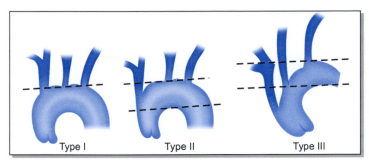

Fig. 5.7: Types of arch of aorta

Arteries of the Head and Neck

Common Carotid Artery

The right common carotid artery arises from the brachiocephalic artery behind the right sternoclavicular joint. The left artery arises from the arch of the aorta in the superior mediastinum.

The common carotid artery runs upward through the neck, diverging laterally from behind the sternoclavicular joint, upto the upper border of the thyroid cartilage. Here, it divides into the external and internal carotid arteries, with a dilatation known as carotid sinus.

Branches

Apart from the two terminal branches, the common carotid artery gives off no branches.

External Carotid Artery

The external carotid artery is one of the terminal branches of the common carotid artery. It supplies structures in the neck, face, and scalp; it also supplies the tongue and the maxilla. The artery begins at the level of the upper border of the thyroid cartilage and terminates in the substance of the parotid gland behind the neck of the mandible by dividing into the superficial temporal and maxillary arteries.

Branches

- Superior thyroid artery, supplies the thyroid gland.
- Ascending pharyngeal artery, supplies the pharyngeal wall.
- Lingual artery, supplies the tongue
- Facial artery, *Branches of the facial artery* supply the tonsil, the submandibular salivary gland, and the muscles and the skin of the face.
- Occipital artery, supplies the back of the scalp
- Posterior auricular artery, supplies the auricle and the scalp
- Superficial temporal artery, supplies the scalp.
- Maxillary artery, with its main branch middle meningeal artery.

Internal Carotid Artery

The internal carotid artery begins at the bifurcation of the common carotid artery at the level of the upper border of the thyroid cartilage. It supplies the brain, the eye, the forehead, and part of the nose, and terminates by dividing into the anterior and the middle cerebral arteries, inside the cranium.

Branches

There are no branches in the neck. Many important branches, however, are given off in the skull.

Ophthalmic Artery

The ophthalmic artery arises from the internal carotid artery. The central artery is an end artery and the only blood supply to the retina.

Posterior Communicating Artery

The posterior communicating artery runs backward to join the posterior cerebral artery.

Anterior Cerebral Artery

The anterior cerebral artery is a terminal branch of the internal carotid artery. It supplies the medial and the superolateral surfaces of the cerebral hemisphere. It is joined to the artery of the opposite side by the *anterior communicating artery*.

Middle Cerebral Artery

The middle cerebral artery is the largest terminal branch of the internal carotid artery. It supplies the entire lateral surface of the cerebral hemisphere except the narrow strip along the superolateral margin (which is supplied by the anterior cerebral artery) and the occipital pole and inferolateral surface of the hemisphere (both of which are supplied by the posterior cerebral artery). The middle cerebral artery thus supplies all the motor area of the cerebral cortex except the leg area. It also gives off central branches that supply central masses of gray matter and the internal capsule of the brain.

Circle of Willis

The circle of Willis lies in the subarachnoid space at the base of the brain. It is formed by the anastomosis between the branches of the two internal carotid arteries and the two vertebral arteries. The anterior communicating, posterior cerebral, and basilar (formed by the junction of the two vertebral arteries) are all arteries that contribute to the circle. Anteriorly, the anterior cerebral arteries of the carotids are joined by the anterior communicating artery. Posteriorly, the basilar artery divides into two posterior cerebral artery, and joined with the ipsilateral internal carotid artery by a posterior communicating artery. Cortical and central branches arise from the circle and supply the brain.

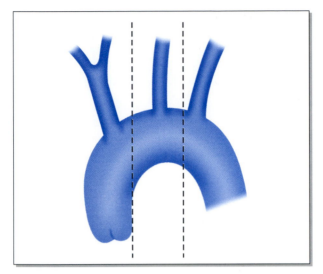

Fig. 5.8: Tracheal air strip

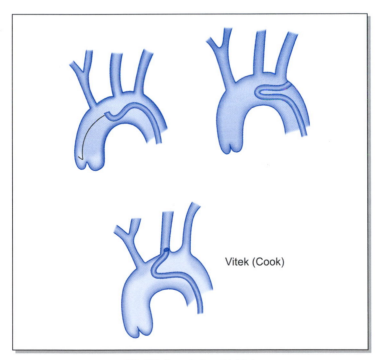

Vitek (Cook)

Fig. 5.9: Cannulation with Vitek

Carotid and cerebral angiography: Start with LAO 40°:
- Tracheal air strip is the marker (Fig. 5.8)
- Innominate artery is on the left, left common carotid artery is middle and left subclavian artery is on the right to the air shadow.

Selective cannulation (Figs 5.9 and 5.10):
- LAO 40° guided by arch anatomy (or tracheal air strip)
- *Simple arch:* Simple catheter (Tables 5.9 and 5.10)

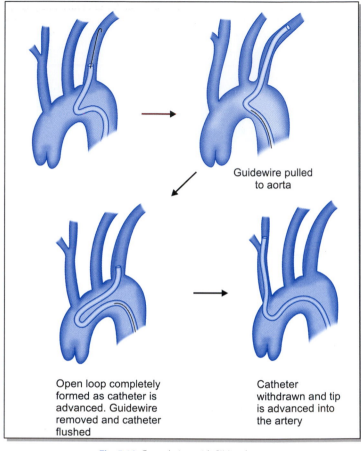

Guidewire pulled
to aorta

Open loop completely
formed as catheter is
advanced. Guidewire
removed and catheter
flushed

Catheter
withdrawn and tip
is advanced into
the artery

Fig. 5.10: Cannulation with SIM catheter

Table 5.9: Catheter selection for carotid angiography

Type of arch	Catheter type	Comments
Simple arch	JR, NTR/3DRC, vertebral, Vitek	Not helpful in complex arch
Complex arch	Vitek	Easy to use, for simple and complex arch. More support
Complex	SIM	Needs to be formed in SCA or aortic root. More support.

- *Complex arch:* Vitek
- Much manipulation is prohibited because of chance of showering of embolus.

Cerebral circulation: Basic views
- AP—Cranial
- Lateral.

Table 5.10: Radiographic view and catheter selection for cerebral angiography

Vessel	Projection	Catheter
Innominate artery	• LAO 30°, • RAO 30° (for bifurcation)	• JR • Vitek
Right common carotid artery	AP, lateral and ipsilateral oblique (RAO)	• JR • Vitek • MP
Right vertebral artery	AP, lateral, RAO	• JR • Vitek • MP
Left common carotid artery—Internal carotid artery	• AP, LAO • AP, RAO • Lateral	• JR • Vitek • MP
Left vertebral artery	• AP, LAO • Lateral	• JR • Vitek • Vertebral

Subclavian Arteries

First part of the subclavian artery: This part gives off the vertebral artery, the thyrocervical trunk, and the internal thoracic artery.

Branches

The *vertebral artery* ascends in the neck through the foramina in the transverse processes of the upper six cervical vertebrae. It passes medially above the posterior arch of the atlas and then ascends through the foramen magnum into the skull. On reaching the anterior surface of the medulla oblongata of the brain at the level of the lower border of the pons, it joins the vessel of the opposite side to form the basilar artery. The *basilar artery* ascends in a groove on the anterior surface of the pons. It gives off branches to the pons, the cerebellum, and the internal ear. It finally divides into the two posterior cerebral arteries. On each side, the *posterior cerebral artery* curves laterally and backward around the midbrain. Cortical branches supply the inferolateral surfaces of the temporal lobe and the visual cortex on the lateral and the medial surfaces of the occipital lobe.

Branches in the neck: Spinal and muscular arteries

Branches in the skull: Meningeal, anterior and posterior spinal, posterior inferior cerebellar, medullary arteries.

The *thyrocervical trunk* is a short trunk that gives off three terminal branches.

1. The *inferior thyroid artery* ascends to the posterior surface of the thyroid gland, where it is closely related to the recurrent laryngeal nerve. It supplies the thyroid and the inferior parathyroid glands.
2. The *superficial cervical artery* is a small branch that crosses the brachial plexus.
3. The *suprascapular artery* runs laterally.

The *internal thoracic (mammary) artery* descends into the thorax behind the 1st costal cartilage and in front of the pleura. in the 6th intercostal space, it divides into the superior epigastric and the musculophrenic arteries. It supplies the upper 6 anterior intercostals spaces through 6 pairs of anterior intercostals arteries.

Second part of the subclavian artery: The second part of the subclavian artery lies behind the scalenus anterior muscle.

Branches: The *costocervical trunk* runs backward over the dome of the pleura and divides into the *superior intercostals artery*, which supplies the 1st and the 2nd intercostals spaces, and the *deep cervical artery*, which supplies the deep muscles of the neck.

Third part of the subclavian artery: The third part of the subclavian artery extends from the lateral border of the scalenus anterior muscle,

Branches: The third part of the subclavian artery usually has no branches.

Axillary Artery

The axillary artery, a continuation of the subclavian artery, begins at the 1st rib's outer border, ending normally at the inferior border of the Teres Major muscle, where it becomes brachial artery.

Branches

1. Superior thoracic
2. Thoraco-acromial
3. Lateral thoracic
4. Subscapular
5. Anterior circumflex humeral
6. Posterior circumflex humeral

Brachial Artery

The brachial artery, a continuation of the axillary artery, begins at the distal (inferior) border of the tendon of teres major and ends about a centimeter distal to the elbow joint (at the level of the neck of the radius). Here it divides into radial and ulnar arteries.

The arteria profunda brachii is a large branch from the postero-medial aspect of the brachial artery. Apart from the muscular rami, it supplies the following branches: the nutrient, deltoid, middle collateral and radial collateral arteries.

Radial Artery

The radial artery, though smaller than the ulnar, appears a more direct continuation of the brachial artery. It continues in the forearm, the wrist and ends in the hand, forming the deep palmar arch.

The deep palmar arch, formed by anastomosis of the end of the radial with the deep palmar branch of the ulnar artery.

Ulnar Artery

The ulnar artery, the larger terminal branch of the brachial artery.

The artery supplies, medial muscles in the forearm and hand, the common flexor synovial sheath and ulnar nerve.

The superficial palmar arch: This anastomosis is fed mainly by the ulnar artery, entering the palm with the ulnar nerve, anterior to the flexor retinaculum. The anastomosis is further completed by the superficial palmar branch of the radial artery.

Descending Thoracic Aorta

The descending thoracic aorta lies in the posterior mediastinum and begins as a continuation of the arch of the aorta on the left side of the lower border of the body of the 4th thoracic vertebra (i.e., opposite the sternal angle). It passes behind the diaphragm (through the aortic opening) in the midline and becomes continuous with the abdominal aorta.

Branches

Posterior intercostal arteries are given off to the lower nine intercostal spaces on each side. *Subcostal arteries* are given off on each side and run along the lower border of the 12th rib to enter the abdominal wall.

Pericardial, esophageal, and *bronchial arteries* are small branches that are distributed to these organs.

Bronchial Arteries (Fig. 5.11)

Bronchial artery angiogram is important for bronchial artery embolization in cases of refractory hemoptysis.

Bronchial arteries commonly originate between T5 and T6.

Bronchial arteries that originate outside T5 and T6 levels are considered to be anomalous or ectopic variants (16–30%). The commonly found variants are of the following types:

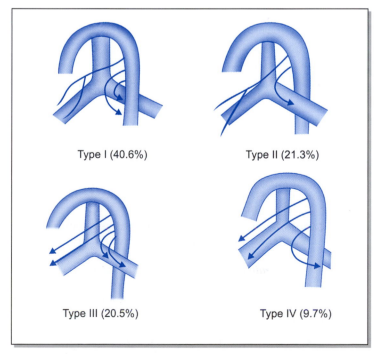

Type I (40.6%)   Type II (21.3%)

Type III (20.5%)   Type IV (9.7%)

Fig. 5.11: Bronchial arteries

- 4–6 bronchial arteries
- Origin from intercostal arteries
- Origin from brachiocephalic trunk
- Origin from subclavian artery
- Origin from thyrocervical trunk
- Origin from internal mammary artery
- Origin from inferior phrenic artery (from abdominal aorta)
- Parasitic arteries.

Bronchial artery angiogram is done by descending thoracic angiography by putting pigtail in LAO view. Selective catheterization requires catheters like cobra, side winder, head hunter, SOS-Omni.

It is important to look for and identification of anterior medullary artery which has a common origin with intercostals arteries and supplies the spinal arteries of thoracic area.

Presence of hair pin loop indicates presence of anterior medullary artery and is a contraindication for embolization. In that case, delivery of embolic agent should be beyond the origin of spinal artery.

Arteries on the Posterior Abdominal Wall

Abdominal Aorta

Location and Description

The aorta enters the abdomen through the aortic opening of the diaphragm in front of the 12th thoracic vertebra. At the level of the 4th lumbar vertebra, it divides into the two common iliac arteries.

Branches

- *Three unpaired ventral branches:* the celiac artery, superior mesenteric artery, and inferior mesenteric artery
- *Four lateral branches:*
  - Inferior phrenic artery, supplies the diaphragm, and gives branch to suprarenal gland.
  - Middle suprarenal artery, opposite the origin of superior mesenteric artery, supplies the suprarenal gland.
  - Renal artery, pair of wide bore arteries, arising at right angle from the aorta just below the superior mesenteric artery, supplying the kidney, pelvis of ureter and renal fat, along with suprarenal gland.
  - Gonadal artery (testicular or ovarian artery). Testicular artery enters the deep inguinal ring and reaches the posterior border of testis and epididymis.
    Ovarian artery enters the broad ligament of uterus, anastomoses with the uterine artery and supplies uterine tube, uterus and ovary.
- *Five dorsal abdominal wall branches:* Four pairs of lumbar arteries and the median sacral artery.
- *Two terminal branches:* The two common iliac arteries.

These branches are summarized in Flow chart 5.1.

Flow chart 5.1: Branches of abdominal aorta

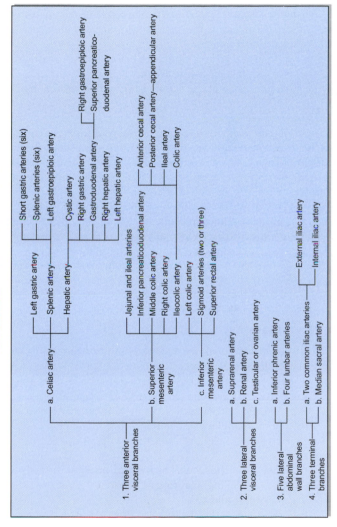

Celiac Trunk

It is a short wide vessel, of about 1.25 cm, which arises from the front of the aorta, immediately below the aortic opening of the diaphragm, opposite the lower border of T_{12} vertebra. The trunk of artery proceeds forward and divides into three branches—*Left gastric, common hepatic* and *splenic*.

The left gastric, the smallest branch, contributes to the stomach through the lesser curvature, along with few ascending esophageal branches.

The common hepatic artery, reaches the right free margin of the lesser omentum, and divides into the *right gastric and gastroduodenal arteries, and the hepatic artery proper*.

The right gastric artery, along the lesser curvature of stomach, anastomoses with the left gastric artery.

The gastroduodenal artery supplies up to the proximal half of first part of duodenum, and divides into *superior pancreaticoduodenal and right gastroepiploic arteries*.

Superior pancreaticoduodenal artery anastomoses with the inferior pancreaticoduodenal artery (branch of superior mesenteric artery).

Right gastroepiploic artery, traverses the greater curvature, supplying the stomach and greater omentum, and anastomosing with the left gastroepiploic artery, branch of splenic artery.

The hepatic artery proper divides into right and left hepatic artery, which supply the physiological right and left lobes of liver, respectively, after division into further segmental branches. The right hepatic artery gives origin to the *cystic artery*, supplying the gallbladder.

The splenic artery is largest and most tortuous branch of the celiac trunk. Before supplying the spleen, it gives origin to *pancreatic, short gastric* (to the fundus) and *left gastroepiploic* arteries.

Superior Mesenteric Artery (Fig. 5.12)

It arises from the front of the aorta, 1 cm below the celiac trunk, opposite the lower border of L_1 vertebra. It supplies the entire small gut, except,

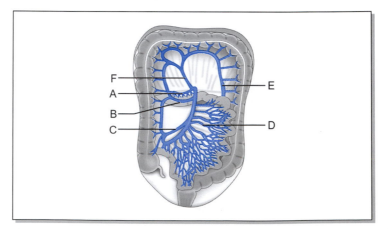

Fig. 5.12: Branches of the superior mesenteric artery (SMA). (A) Inferior pancreaticoduodenal artery; (B) Right colic artery; (C) Ileocolic artery; (D) Jejunal and ileal branches; (E) Marginal artery of drummond; (F) Middle colic artery

the proximal part of the duodenum up to the ampulla of Vater, and also supplies the large gut, upto the junction of the right two-third and left one-third of the transverse colon. In addition, it supplies a part of the pancreatic head.

Major Branches

12–15 jejunal and ileal branches, which pass between layers of mesentery and form series of arches.

Inferior pancreaticoduodenal artery, arising as the first branch, anastomoses with superior pancreaticoduodenal artery.

Middle colic artery, originates from superior mesenteric artery, at the lower border of the pancreas, and enters the root of transverse mesocolon. It divides into right and left branches. The right branch reaches the right colic flexure and anastomoses with the ascending branch of right colic artery; the left branch anastomoses close to the left colic flexure with the left colic branch of inferior mesenteric artery.

Right colic artery, reaches the ascending colon and divides into ascending and descending branches, to anastomose respectively with the middle colic and ascending branch of ileocolic arteries, respectively.

Ileocolic artery, terminal branch, reaches the right iliac fossa and divides into ascending and descending branches. The ascending branch anastomoses with the right colic artery. The descending branch divides into four sets of branches—anterior and posterior cecal, appendicular and ileal arteries.

Inferior Mesenteric Artery (Fig. 5.13)

It arises from the front of the aorta about 4 cm, above the aortic bifurcation, opposite the L_3 vertebra.

It supplies the left one-third of the transverse colon, the entire descending colon, and sigmoid colon, the rectum, and the upper part of the anal canal upto the pectinate line.

It gives off the *left colic artery, two or three sigmoid arteries* and continues as the *superior rectal artery*.

The left colic artery reaches the left colic flexure, and divides into the ascending and descending branches. The former anastomoses with the

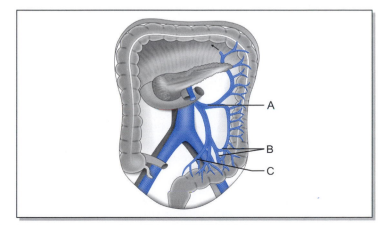

Fig. 5.13: Branches of the IMA (inferior mesenteric artery). (A) Left colic artery; (B) Sigmoid arteries; (C) Superior rectal arteries

middle colic artery after entering the transverse mesocolon; while the latter anastomoses with the highest sigmoid artery.

Peculiarities

The successive anastomoses of colic branches of the superior and inferior mesenteric arteries form a continuous *marginal artery of Drummond* which extends from the ileocecal to the rectosigmoid junction. Straight vesssels arising from the marginal artery supply the large gut by dividing into longer and shorter branches.

Critical point of Sudeck: Point of origin of the last sigmoid branch originating from the inferior mesenteric artery. It is essential to retain this critical point during colorectal surgery as removal may lead to ischemia of the colon. This is particularly true when the anastomosis of superior rectal artery and last sigmoid branch of inferior mesenteric artery is deficient and ligation of superior rectal artery may lead to ischemia of proximal stump.

In few cases, the anastomosis between the middle colic and the left colic arteries does not exist. In such condition, a direct retroperitoneal anastomotic arcade, *the arc of Riolan*, is observed between the trunks of superior and inferior mesenteric arteries.

Gastrointestinal Angiography

Any angiographic evaluation of a patient with acute gastrointestinal bleeding should begin with selective catheterization of the artery supplying the most likely site of bleeding as determined by the available clinical, endoscopic and imaging data.

In suspected upper gastrointestinal hemorrhage, celiac artery evaluation should be done first, followed by superior mesenteric artery (SMA) as the latter may contribute to a site of upper gastrointestinal bleeding through pancreaticoduodenal arcade.

In suspected lower gastrointestinal bleeding, SMA should be first evaluated. It supplies small bowel and a part of the large gut up to transverse colon. Inferior mesenteric artery (IMA) supplies large gut from transverse colon to rectum and anal canal. The lower part is also supplied by branches of internal iliac arteries and this may become a dominant vascular pattern, when IMA gets blocked, and thus supply the entire large gut via the arc of Riolan or the marginal artery of Drummond.

Selective Cannulation (Fig. 5.14)

Common Iliac Arteries

The right and left common iliac arteries are the terminal branches of the aorta. They arise at the level of the 4th lumbar vertebra and run downward. Each artery ends in front of the sacroiliac joint by dividing into the external and internal iliac arteries.

External Iliac Artery

It gives off the *inferior epigastric* and *deep circumflex iliac* branches.

The artery enters the thigh by passing under the inguinal ligament to become the femoral artery. The inferior epigastric artery arises just

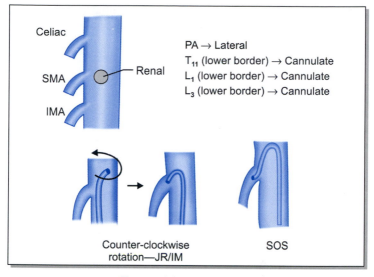

Fig. 5.14: Selective cannulation

above the inguinal ligament. It passes upward and medially along the medial margin of the deep inguinal ring and enters the rectus sheath behind the rectus abdominis muscle.

The deep circumflex iliac artery arises close to the inferior epigastric artery. It ascends laterally to the anterior superior iliac spine and the iliac crest, supplying the muscles of the anterior abdominal wall.

Femoral Artery

The femoral artery, a continuation of the external iliac artery, begins behind the inguinal ligament, midway between the anterior superior iliac spine and the symphysis pubis, descends the thigh anteromedially and becomes the popliteal artery as it passes through an opening in the adductor magnus, near the junction of the middle and distal thirds of the thigh. Proximally it is in the femoral triangle, and distally in the adductor (subsartorial) canal.

Branches

- *The superficial epigastric artery* arises anteriorly, from the femoral artery, about 1 cm distal to the inguinal ligament. It ascends anterior to the ligament and runs in the abdominal superficial fascia, almost to the umbilicus. It anastomoses with the branches of the inferior epigastric.
- *The superficial circumflex iliac artery*, arises near or with the superficial epigastric. It runs laterally distal to the inguinal ligament towards the anterior superior iliac spine. It supplies the skin, superficial fascia and superficial inguinal lymph nodes, anastomosing with the deep circumflex iliac, superior gluteal and lateral circumflex femoral arteries.
- *The superficial external pudendal artery* arises medially from the femoral, close to the preceding branches. It passes medially

to supply the lower abdominal, penile, scrotal or labial skin, anastomosing with branches of the internal pudendal.

- *The deep external pudendal artery*, passes medially, to supply the skin of the perineum and scrotum or labium majus.

Muscular Branches

- *Arteria profunda femoris (Deep femoral artery):* Discussed below.
- *The descending genicular artery*
- *The popliteal artery (Terminal branch)*

The *arteria profunda femoris:* This large branch arises laterally, from the femoral artery, about 3.5 cm distal to the inguinal ligament. The deep femoral artery is the main supply to the adductor, flexor and extensor muscles. It also anastomoses with the internal and external iliac arteries above and the popliteal artery below.

The popliteal artery: A continuation of the femoral artery, traverses the popliteal fossa. It descends laterally, inclining obliquely to the distal border of the popliteus, where it divides into the anterior and posterior tibial arteries.

The Arteria Dorsalis Pedis

The continuation of the anterior tibial artery to the ankle and dorsum of foot, complete the plantar arch, where it provides the 1st plantar metatarsal artery.

Branches

Tarsal, arcuate and 1st dorsal metatarsal arteries.

The Posterior Tibial Artery

This begins at the distal border of the popliteus, descending medially in the flexor compartment.

Branches

Circumflex fibular, peroneal, nutrient, medial and lateral plantar arteries.

The plantar arch: This is deeply situated, extending from the 5th metatarsal base to the proximal end of the 1st interosseous space.

Internal Iliac Artery

The internal iliac artery passes down into the pelvis in front of the sacroiliac joint.

Arteries of the True Pelvis

The following arteries enter the pelvic cavity:

- Internal iliac artery
- Superior rectal artery
- Ovarian artery
- Median sacral artery.

Internal Iliac Artery

The internal iliac artery passes down into the pelvis to the upper margin of the greater sciatic foramen, where it divides into anterior and posterior divisions.

Major Branches of the Anterior Division (Fig. 5.15)

- *Umbilical artery:* From the proximal patent part of the umbilical artery arises the *superior vesical artery*, which supplies the upper portion of the bladder
- *Obturator artery:* This artery runs forward along the lateral wall of the pelvis with the obturator nerve and leaves the pelvis through the obturator canal.
- *Inferior vesical artery:* This artery supplies the base of the bladder and the prostate and seminal vesicles in the male; it also gives off the *artery to the vas deferens.*
- *Middle rectal artery:* Commonly, this artery arises with the inferior vesical artery. It supplies the muscle of the lower rectum and anastomoses with the superior rectal and inferior rectal arteries.
- *Internal pudendal artery:* Its branches supply the musculature of the anal canal and the skin and muscles of the perineum.
- *Inferior gluteal artery*
- *Uterine artery:* It supplies the ovary, uterus and vagina by anastomoses with the ovarian artery and vaginal artery.

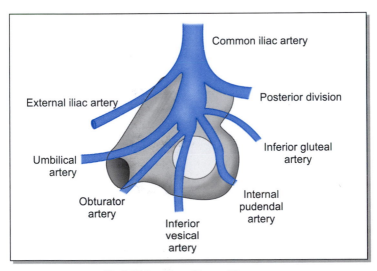

Fig. 5.15: Branches of internal iliac artery:
Ipsilateral oblique 35°–40° with 10°–15° cranial/caudal

- Prostatic artery usually comes out of superior vesical artery, while uterine artery comes out from inferior vesical artery
- Internal iliac artery can be cannulated from opposite side (IMA catheter) and from the same side with SIM catheter

Suggested Reading

1. Assessment of Coronary Calcification by Angiography: Yoshinobu Onua–SPIRIT-II Study Catheter Cardiovascular Intervention. 2010;76:634-42.
2. Clauk J. Procedural techniques of Coronary Angiography: www.Intechopen.com.
3. Percutaneous Coronary Intervention versus Coronary Artery Bypass Grafting for Severe Coronary Artery Disease (The SYNTAX Trial): N Eng J Med. 2009;360:961-72.
4. TIMI—Definitions: www. TIMI.org Coronary Ectasia: Diagnosis and Treatment: Maurogenis—E-Journal of Cardiogenic Practice Vol. 8, ESC 2009.

Guide Catheters
(The Platform)

- Shuvanan Ray

The most under-rated asset to coronary angioplasty that prevented launch of PTCA on March 22, 1976—(Bernherd Meier; 2005).

Guide Catheter

It is basically a conduit for delivery and support for
- Contrast
- Wire
- Device (i.e. stents, balloons)

Structural differences make guide catheters more stiff, having less torque control and more liable to be kinked than diagnostic catheters. So respond differently to manipulation than diagnostic catheter (Table 6.1).

Guide catheters are placed in the aorta to enter the coronary ostium by its tip and provide support, so that interventional devices can be passed through it without displacing the guide catheter from the ostium.

Table 6.1: Guide catheter and diagnostic catheter (Fig. 6.1)

Diagnostic catheter	Guide catheter
Thicker wall yet less radial strength	Thinner wall with greater radial strength
Lumen, narrower	Wider
Round wire braid pattern layered between inner and outer jackets	Encapsulated flat wire braid enables thinner robust walls without compromising support
Tapered tip, tighter primary curve	Nontappered shorter tip and more open primary curve
Made from one mandrel	Constituted by fusion of 3–5 segments (like a soft tip, a torque zone and a support zone and shaft) made separately

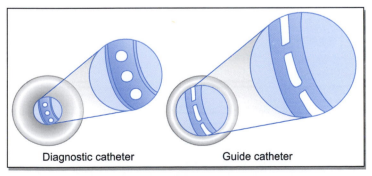

Diagnostic catheter   Guide catheter

Fig. 6.1: Cross-section of guide and diagnostic catheters

The support can be obtained from the shape of guide catheter and its contact with the opposite aortic wall. On the other hand, support can be obtained by manipulating the guide catheter deep inside the artery (deep seating).

Depending on the Support, Classificatin of Guide Catheters (Flow chart 6.1, Table 6.2)

Active Support

Use the artery itself to ensure guide curve conformability and back up (deep seating) and relies on active manipulation of guiding catheter to obtain stable position, seat coaxially.

Passive Support

Relies on properties of the shaft and tip to maintain position in the ostium and depends on support by either anatomy or catheter composition, curve or shape. Active manipulation not possible (prefer minimal manipulation.

Balanced Support

Rely on properties of the shaft and tip to maintain position in the ostium but prefer a flexible distal segment that can be manipulated/seated for extra backup if needed.

Runway catheters: An excellent group of catheters have been introduced recently (Boston Scientific). The catheters are three layered:
1. Innermost layer of PTFE
2. Metal shaft with stainless steel wire braids
3. Outermost coat of polyurethane

Flow chart 6.1: Choosing types of support

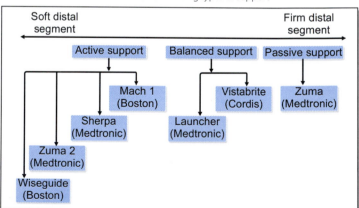

Table 6.2: Basic characters of different support guide cath

Guide catheter	Requires precise curve selection and sizing	Requires large ostium	Requires disease-free ostium
Active support	No	Yes	Yes
Balanced support	No	Indeterminate	Indeterminate
Passive support	Yes	Indeterminate	Indeterminate

They are 6F catheters with an inner diameter of 0.70 inch. They are kink resistant and highly torque able. Many more shapes have been introduced and they are equally effective both from radial and femoral access and can be deep throttled because of soft, atraumatic tip.

Basic Shapes of Guide Catheters

There are almost 250 shapes of guide catheter available, most of which are not really necessary in day-to-day practice. Only three shapes (Judkin's, Amplatz and extra backup) are essential to know and in almost all cases, they will be successful for conducting the procedure. There are one or two special catheters which are occasionally used in very special situations like anomalous origin, postcoronary artery bypass grafting cases and should be kept in the shelf (like LIMA, multipurpose, MAC) and for radial PCI (MUTA and Ikari).

Basic Guiding Catheter Selection

It depends on three important factors:
1. Size
2. Curve
3. Special characters

Size: In most cases 6F or 7F catheters are all that it necessary for performing the procedure safely. Most guide catheter in 6F has an internal diameter > 0.7 inch and 7F > 0.80 inch. Routine angioplasties can be done easily with 6F guide catheter but complex angioplasties requiring two stents or rotablation with burr > 1.5 requires 7F guide catheter.

Curve: Mostly used catheters are either Judkin's and extra backup catheters. The size (3, 3.5 or 4) depends upon the distance between the primary and secondary curve (Figs 6.2A and B).

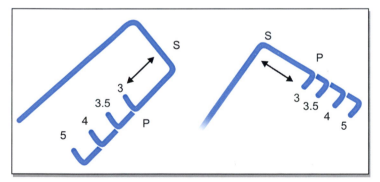

Fig. 6.2A: Judkins left catheter
Abbreviations: P, primary curve; S, secondary curve

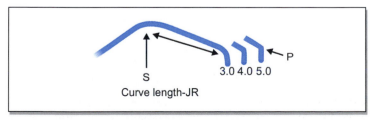

Fig. 6.2B: Judkins right catheter

Depending on width an aorta may be narrow, normal, or dilated/elongated (Fig. 6.3).

The left coronary artery (Fig. 6.4) originates from the middle portion of the left coronary sinus, just inferior to the sinotubular junction and the proximal segment of the artery pursues an orthogonal course with respect to the sinus. Similarly, ostium of the right coronary artery (Fig. 6.5) generally arises from middle of the coronary sinus, just inferior to sinotubular junction and again the proximal part takes an orthogonal course with respect to sinus. The cannulation of LCA and RCA in different anatomy is shown in Figs 6.6 to 6.8.

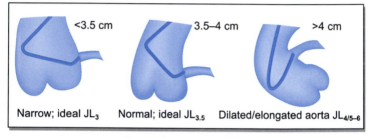

Fig. 6.3: Cannulation with JL$_{3.5}$

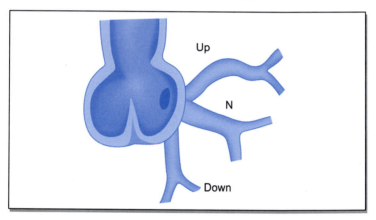

Fig. 6.4: Left coronary artery—origin and trajectory

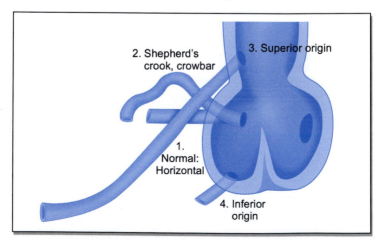

Fig. 6.5: Right coronary artery—origin and trajectory

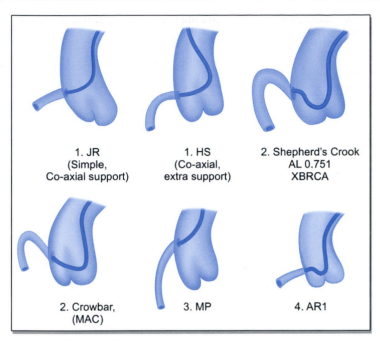

Fig. 6.6: RCA cannulation according to origin and trajectory

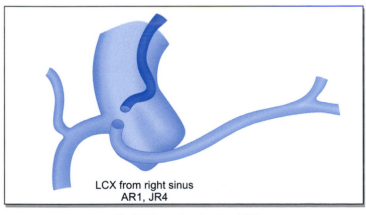

Fig. 6.7: Anomalously arising LCX

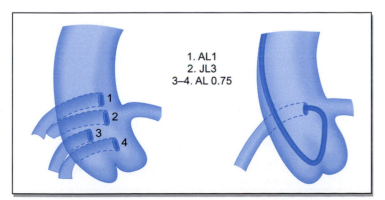

Fig. 6.8: Anomalously arising RCA

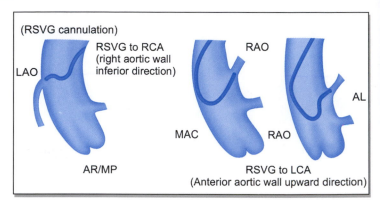

Fig. 6.9: Reversed saphenous vein grafting (RSVG) cannulation
Abbreviations: RAO, radial artery occlusion; LAO, left anterior oblique; LCA, left coronary artery; RCA, right coronary artery; MAC, mitral annular calcification

Similarly, the venous grafts cannulation requires different catheters according to their position, and is shown in Fig. 6.9.

Cannulation of Coronary Arteries

Two very important facts are to be remembered during guide selection:
1. **Origin:** Whether the artery is arising from the normal site (variations are: high, low, anterior and posterior)
2. **Trajectory:** Horizontal, upward or downward

Length of the proximal segment of the artery often demands an increased back-up support of the guide catheter.

Pressure Dumping or Proximal Lesions

When the guide catheter occludes the coronary artery, there is a change in the arterial pressure waveforms into more of a square wave pattern called 'damping' or ventricularization. This indicates significant obstruction to flow or no coaxial orientation of the guide tip.

A guide catheter with small holes near the tip (sidehole catheter) reduce ischemia when catheter is seated in a small artery. However, sideholes may lead to inadequate artery visualization and contrast loss and actually the pressure reflected through guiding catheter is the aortic pressure now giving a false sense of security while coronary flow is still reduced.

For Asian patients with normal aortic route (3.5 cm) a JL 3.5 (Judkins) usually fits well, superior trajectory of LAD or narrow aortic root—smaller size (JL 3) guide is necessary. Horizontal or wide aortic root – JL with long secondary curve (5 or 6) will be required.

Checking Stability and Back-up (Figs 6.10 to 6.13)

Push test: Forward advancement of the guide should further intubate the coronary artery rather than prolapse into aortic root.

If tip slips out: Guide does not provide sufficient back-up, it means to be changed for another with better support.

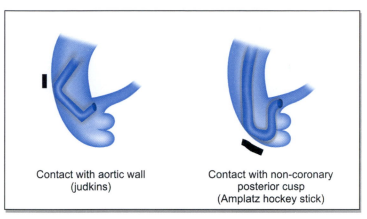

Contact with aortic wall
(judkins)

Contact with non-coronary
posterior cusp
(Amplatz hockey stick)

Fig. 6.10: Back-up support

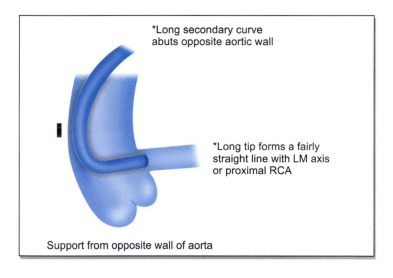

*Long secondary curve
abuts opposite aortic wall

*Long tip forms a fairly
straight line with LM axis
or proximal RCA

Support from opposite wall of aorta

Fig. 6.11: Extra back-up support

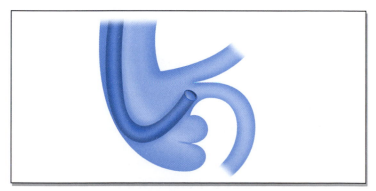

Fig. 6.12: Tip of guide is very close to the ostium of LcX. Acuity of LM and LcX angle nullified, making smoother transition between LM and LcX

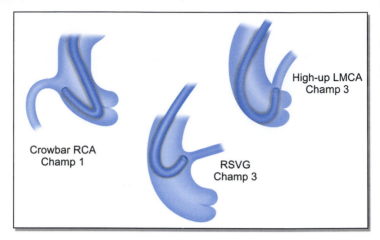

Fig. 6.13: Superior oriented arteries and saphenous vein grafts

When better back-up support catheter is not available or not fitting following techniques to be followed to stabilize the guide:

- Deep throttling
- Buddy wire
- Second wire in a side branch (anchor wire)
- Anchor balloon (1.5 – 2 mm balloon)
- Mother and child (inserted in a small proximal branch @ 2 atm)
- Long sheath

Guide Cath Selection: An Algorithm (Flow chart 6.2)

Flow chart 6.2: Guide catheter selection

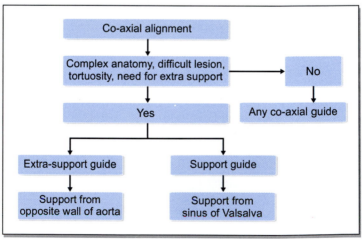

Contd...

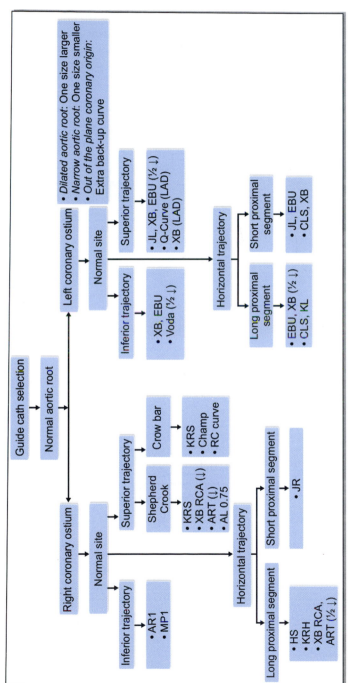

Contd...

Guide Catheter Manipulation from Radial Access

Manipulation of guide catheter from radial side is not different from that though femoral access when ascending aorta is vertical. In obese or severely hypertensive patients who have a horizontal aorta the difference is more marked and makes manipulation difficult—in such aorta, the catheter (either from right or left radial) will approach the coronary artery from left side and cannulation of LCA and support will become a clinical issue (Fig. 6.14).

Transradial Guiding Catheter Shape Selection

	Left coronary artery	Right coronary artery
Left radial	Standard catheters	
Right radial	XB, EBU, Voda (↓0.5)	JR (↑0.5)
	IKARI left	Amplatz R/L
	CLS, Q-curve	IKARI left or right (Fig. 6.15)
		KRH, KRS, RC, XBRCA

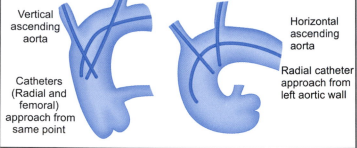

Fig. 6.14: Comparison of catheter position from radial and femoral in normal and abnormal aorta

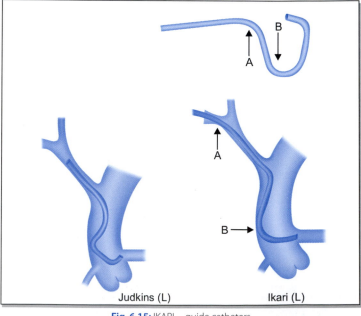

Fig. 6.15: IKARI—guide catheters

Benefits of IKARI Catheter

- Can be used as JL catheter
- When pushed, tip does not move forward but assumes a power position by abutting to the opposite aortic wall
- Ostial dissection is rare

General rules for radial route: Usually JL/extra backup, take one size smaller than femoral cannulation (based on width of aorta) (Fig. 6.16).

Special techniques for difficult cases—obtaining active back-up by deep seating (Fig. 6.17).

Deep Throttling (Fig. 6.18)

- Judkins or EBU catheter to be used
- Proximal coronary artery diameter should be bigger than the catheter
- Proximal coronary artery should be disease-free
- Always done over a balloon
- Amplatz catheters generally are not be used for deep seating
- *Procedure:* Open the TB valve
- Put the balloon in the artery and inflate at 6–8 atmosphere pressure
- Pull the balloon while rotate and push the catheter, it will go in.

Amplatzing: Over an inflated balloon a Judkins catheter may be rotated and pushed to have support from the opposite wall (Fig. 6.19).

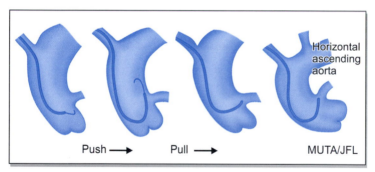

Fig. 6.16: MUTA and JFL catheter manipulation from right radial route

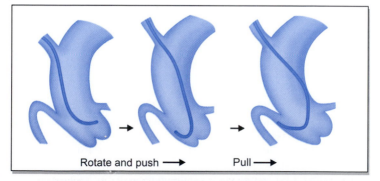

Fig. 6.17: Cannulation of Shepherd's Crook RCA with MAC catheter

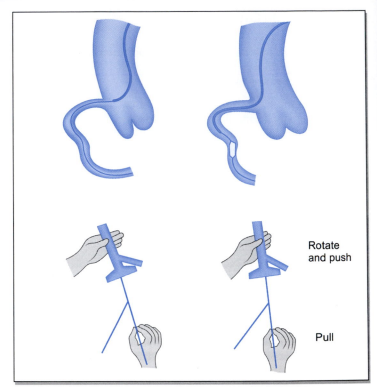

Fig. 6.18: Deep throttling

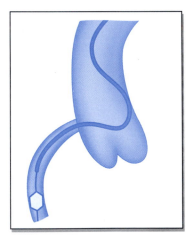

Fig. 6.19: Amplatzing of JR guide catheter

Guide Catheter Extension

GuideLiner and Guidezilla: The extension guide cath (Rapid exchange section—20 cm) (Fig. 6.20)

- Guideliner is a flexible, 20 cm straight, soft-tipped extension tube, which is silicon coated
- The catheter is introduced as a balloon through the Y connector

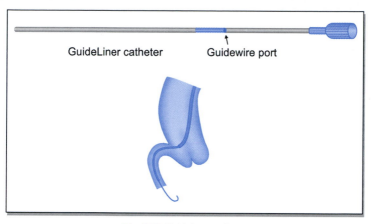

Fig. 6.20: GuideLiner catheter

Table 6.3: Guidezilla versus GuideLiner

	Guidezilla	*GuideLiner*
Size	6F (1.7 mm)	6F (1.78 mm)
Proximal shaft	Stainless steel hypotube	Stainless steel ribbon
Coatup	Hydrophilic (Bioslide)	Silicon wipe
ID	0.057 inch	0.056 inch
OD	0.066 inch	0.067 inch
Distal guide length	25 cm	25 cm

- The catheter is passed on the wire as a rapid exchange balloon deep inside the artery
- Reduces the inner diameter of motherguide by 1 Fr but provides extrasupport to deliver stent in tortuous anatomy (Table 6.3).

Suggested Reading

1. de Man FH, Tandjung K, Hartmann M, et al. Usefulness and safety of the GuideLiner catheter to enhance intubation and support of guide catheters: Insight from the Twente GuideLiner registry. Eurointervention. 2012;8(3):336-44.
2. Frits Haf de Man, Kenneth Tandjung, Marc Hartman. Eurointervention. 2012;8:336-44.
3. IP Cassely, JC Messenger. Catheters and techniques. Cardiol Clin. 2009;27: 417-32.
4. Masahiko Ochiai. Guiding Catheter Back-up for Complex cases. Catheter Cardiovascular Intervention.
5. Nguyen et. Al. Advanced interventional cardiology—Tips and Tricks. Willey-Blackwell, 2013.

7

CHAPTER

Guidewires
(The Lifeline)

■ Shuvanan Ray

Guidewire is passed across the atheromatous block more by application of judgment than of force. — **Dotter and Judkins**

Guidewire selection is a mandatory component of successful coronary intervention. It provides a platform for subsequent delivery of balloon catheter, stents or other devices, so guidewires have following functions:
- To track through the vessel
- To access the lesion
- To cross the lesion atraumatically
- To provide support for interventional devices.

Structure of Guidewire

Any guidewire has six basic components (Fig. 7.1):
1. Core material
2. Core diameter
3. Core taper and grind
4. Tip design
5. Coils and coverings
6. Coatings

Core: The inner part of the guidewire is referred to as core. It extends from proximal to distal part where it begins to taper. The core material provides:
1. Steerability and trackability
2. Flexibility
3. Support of guidewire.

Core diameter influences:
- Flexibility
- Support
- Torque of the wire.

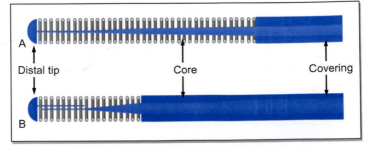

Fig. 7.1: Three components of a guidewire

1. Core material may be stainless steel, nitinol or other alloys. Stainless steel provides excellent support and transmission of torque and push but less flexibility than newer core materials.

   Nitinol is a superelastic kink resistant alloy. It provides excellent flexibility and steering, and retains its shape excellently to be used to treat multiple lesions with tortuosity but is less torquable.

2. Core diameter and core taper are two important parameters which provide pushability, torque transmission and support of guidewires.

3. *Core taper:* The part of the wire where the diameter of the core changes over a set distance.

   Core grind: The part of the core with constant diameter.

   Broad, gradual or long tapers offer acute vessel access and improved tracking. The wire follows itself well-around bends. While, abrupt or short tapers create support (Fig. 7.2).

   Larger diameter, short taper are strong wires with very good support, sometimes needed to deliver bulky devices. On the other hand, smaller diameter and larger taper provides excellent flexibility.

4. *Distal tip:* Function of the tip is to navigate across the difficult anatomy, which may be a stenosed segment, tortuous or angled segment or altogether. The distal tip of a guidewire is usually of two types:

   i. *Core to tip design:* Here the core extends all the way to the tip where it tapers to a variable extent. These wires have precise steering and tip control and a necessary stiffness for crossing resistant lesions.

   ii. *Shaping ribbon design:* Here the core stops just short of distal tip. A small piece of metal (a shaping ribbon) bridges the gap between the end of the core and distal tip. This makes the tip very flexible, soft, easy shaping and good shape retention property. These wires are mainly floaters. They float with the flow and cross the lesion. They are atraumatic and are used in crossing dissected segments.

   Tip design affects steering and durability, and is also responsible for penetration power of the tip.

   Penetration power = Tip stiffness ÷ Area of guidewire tip (Fig. 7.3)

   $$[\text{Penetration power} = 0.004 \text{ kg}/(3.14 * 0.006^2) \text{ kg/inch}^2$$
   $$= 40 \text{ kg/inch}^2]$$

5. *Coils and Coverings:*

   Spring tip coils: Coils affect support, steering, tracking and visibility as well as tactile feedback. They also facilitate shaping and shape retention. Core to tip wires were initially difficult to shape and even after shaping the shape retention was poor. With newer wires

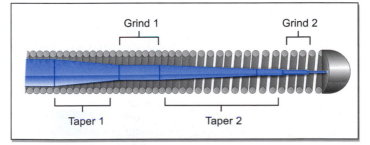

Fig. 7.2: Core taper and core grind

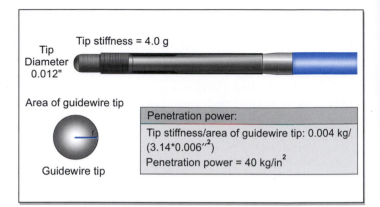

Fig. 7.3: Penetration power versus tip area

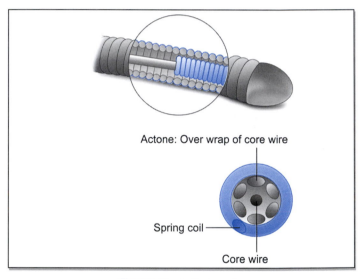

Fig. 7.4: Composite core wire

(ASHAHI), insertion of jointless platinum to stainless spring coils, there is increased torquability, flexibility and resiliency of the tip to core wires.

The new wires of ASHAHI (GAIA, Fielder-XT, R-SION) contain another wire coil at the tip (Rope coils) which enable the wires to have excellent torque control without whip movement and particularly helpful in chronic total occlusion (CTO) crossing (Figs 7.4 and 7.5). *Guidewire covers:* Some guidewires are covered distally with polymer or plastic. This polymer jacket provides lubricity to the wire and allows smooth tracking through tortuosity. Polymer jacketed wires lose tactile feedbacks, and can easily go into subintimal spaces or perforate.

6. *Coatings:* Some wires have hydrophilic coating on their outer surface. This coating minimizes friction and provides better trackability. The hydrophilic coating attracts water to create a gel like surface (Fig. 7.6).

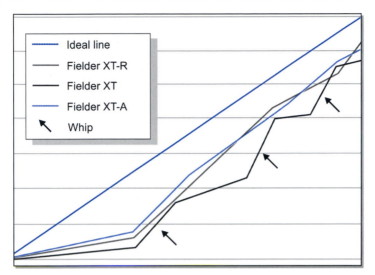

Fig. 7.5: Whip movement during torque

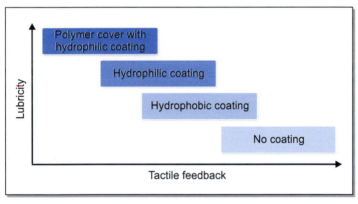

Fig. 7.6: Coating and lubricity of the guidewire

Working classification of guidewires (Table 7.1):
Tip load classified the wire into floppy, intermediate and standard. Floppy wires are better to seek and cross the lesion (side branch access, fine tortuous channels and microchannels) without penetrative force (Flow charts 7.1 and 7.2). Intermediate and standard wires have more penetrative power and usually used in tough lesions and CTOs.

Special Guidewires According to Tip Load

Tip load scale is a test designed to measure a wire's tip stiffness when a bending force required to deflect the tip 2 mm when the wire is braced 10 mm from the tip (Flow chart 7.3).

Table 7.1: Classification of the wires

Criteria	Categorization
Construction material	1. Stainless steel 2. Nitinol 3. High tensile strength stainless steel 4. Hybrid
Tip style	1. Core to tip design (one piece) 2. Shaping ribbon design (2 piece)
Tip cover	1. Spring coil 2. Polymer/plastic cover 3. Micro-cut nitinol sleeve
Coating	1. Hydrophilic (entire working length including tip coils) 2. Hydrophobic (silicon coat on working length except tip)
Tip tapering	1. Non-tapered tip 2. Tapered tip
Tip flexibility	1. Floppy 2. Intermediate 3. Standard/Stiff
Device support	1. Light support 2. Moderate support 3. Extra support

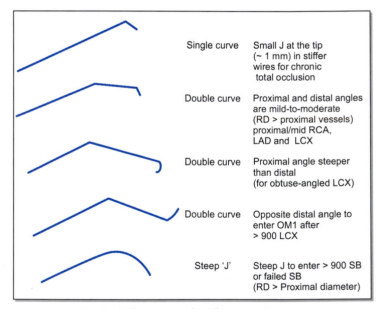

Fig. 7.7: Different shapes for different vessel patterns

Manipulation of Guidewire

Actual manipulation is two-step process:

Shaping of the wire (Figs 7.7 and 7.8): A bent at the tip of the wire allows it to be manipulated. One of the fundamental functions of the steerable J wire is its ability to deviate from the direct pathway, the major determinant of this function is the perpendicular distance of the tip of the wire created by the curve, to the longitudinal axis of the wire. This may be designated as reaching distance (RD) (Fig. 7.9).

Flow chart 7.1: Floppy guidewires

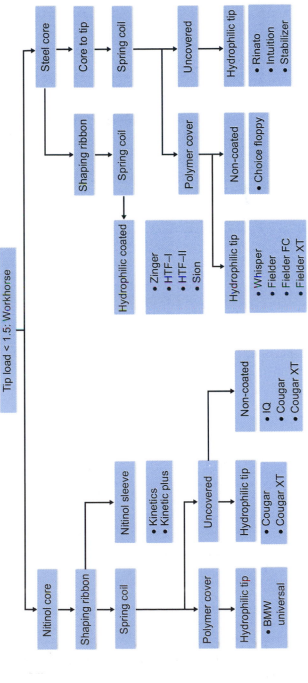

Tip load < 1.5: Workhorse

Run-through:
- Proximal Steel, distal Nitinol
- Shaping ribbon, hydrophilic coated

Steel core → Core to tip → Spring coil

Shaping ribbon → Spring coil

Hydrophilic coated
- Zinger
- HTF-I
- HTF-II
- Sion

Uncovered

Hydrophilic tip
- Rinato
- Intuition
- Stabilizer

Polymer cover

Non-coated
- Choice floppy

Hydrophilic tip
- Whisper
- Fielder
- Fielder FC
- Fielder XT

Nitinol core → Shaping ribbon → Spring coil

Nitinol sleeve
- Kinetics
- Kinetic plus

Uncovered

Non-coated
- IQ
- Cougar
- Cougar XT

Hydrophilic tip
- Cougar
- Cougar XT

Polymer cover

Hydrophilic tip
- BMW
  universal

Flow chart 7.2: Special guidewires (tortuous, calcified, subtotal chronic total occlusion)

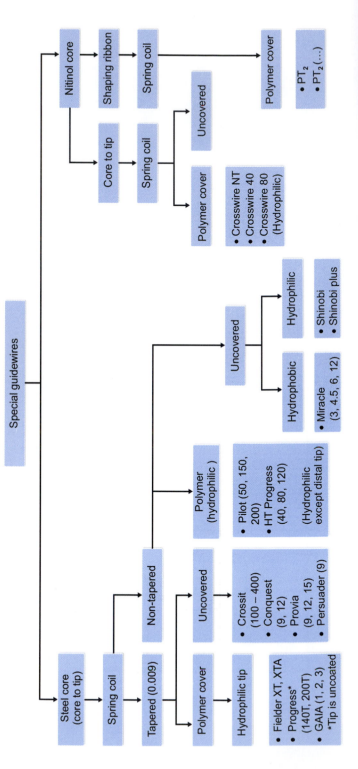

Flow chart 7.3: Speical guidewire according to tip load

Specialty guidewires

Polymer covered hydrophilic		
Wire	Tip diameter	Tip stiffness
•Fielder XT	0.009	1.2 g
PILOT 50	0.014	1.5 g
PILOT 150, 200	0.014	2.7, 4.1 g
Choice PT	0.014	1.9 g
PT Graphics, PT2	0.014	2.6–3.1 g
Shinobi	0.014	7 g
Shinobi Plus	0.014	7 g
Progress 40, 80, 120	0.012	4.8, 9.7, 13 g
Progress 140T, 200T	0.010, 0.009	12.5, 13 g

Non-covered coil wire		
Wire	Tip diameter	Tip stiffness
Crossit 100 XT	0.010	1.7 g
Miraclebros	0.014	3.9, 4.4, 8.8, 13 g
Conquest	0.009	8.6 g
Conquest-Pro	0.009	9.3, 12.4 g
Persuader 3, 6	0.014	5.1, 8 g
Persuader 9	0.011	9.1 g

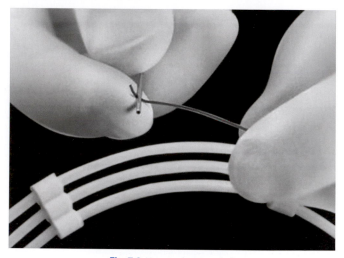

Fig. 7.8: How to shape a wire?

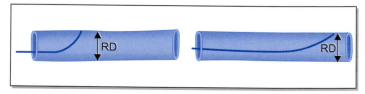

Fig. 7.9: Steeper angle or longer arm have same reaching distance (RD)

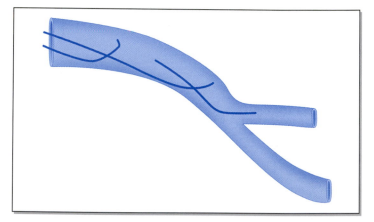

Fig. 7.10: Behavior of reaching distance (RD) in large artery and side branch

Reaching distance, if larger than the diameter of the artery helps wire to enter the side branch.

Reaching distance is flattened when diameter of the vessel is smaller but enters side branch easily when reaching distance opened at the origin of side branch (Fig. 7.10).

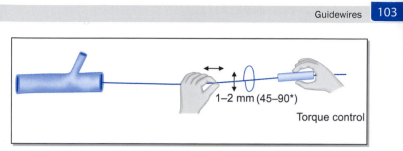

Fig. 7.11: Steering wire through a vessel

Steering of the wire through the vessel (Fig. 7.11):
Use both hands, one hand to steer and another to perform—small alternating rotations by the torque to the left or right, so that the wire does not pick side branches or plaque.

Special Situations

Difficult Side Branch Wirings

Predictors of difficult side branch (SB) wirings are:
1. Severe calcifications involving proximal MV and/or ostium of SB
2. Severe stenosis with a large plaque burden in proximal MV
3. Tortuosity of the proximal MV limiting guidewire manipulations
4. Severe stenosis of SB ostium (< TIMI-3)
5. Distal bifurcation angle > 70° (especially > 90°)
6. Compromised SB flow after MV Stenting.

In a very tight SB lesion or with SB take off > 90°, there are two techniques:
1. Double curved wire
2. Antegrade pushing (Fig. 7.12)/pull-back wiring.

Pull-back wiring: To be tied in Medina 1:1:1 with an unfavorable angle of 90°, a guidewire that has been smoothly curved to shape a broad distal bend is advanced in the distal main vessel where it is pulled back towards the bifurcation. Owing to the hook-like bend the distal tip of the guidewire engages the SB (Fig. 7.13).

Reverse wiring: To be tied in Medina 0:0:1 with extreme angulation (150°) of the SB. A guidewire with a hair pin bend at about 3–5 cm from its distal tip is advanced in the MB, then the guidewire is pulled back from distal MB towards the bifurcation. Owing to the straight bend, the distal tip engages the SB, then gentle turning counter-clockwise advances the guidewire in the SB (Fig. 7.14).

A plastic jacket hydrophilic wire is reasonable for the procedure, because they offer both good controllability for engaging the ostium of extremely angulated branches and better trackability for advancement deep into the vessel because of lower resistance, even under condition of poor push-ability.

Once the tip engages the ostium of the branch, pulling the guidewire back forces the tip to advance into the distal vessel until the bend in the hairpin reaches the bifurcation, application of a gentle forward force with adequate rotation on the shaft allows the tip to advance further into the vessel.

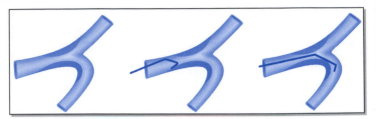

Fig. 7.12: Antegrade pushing

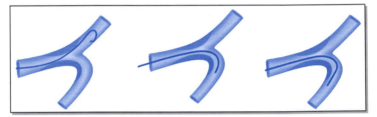

Fig. 7.13: Pull-back wiring

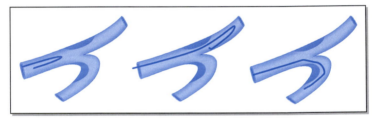

Fig. 7.14: Reverse wiring

Re-entering a Stent

To re-enter a deployed stent sometimes become difficult, as the wire could enter through or in-between struts. In this case to move a balloon or device will be difficult or may destabilize the stent.

Take a workhorse wire, ideally non-coated, make a large curve, cross with a loop (Fig. 7.15).

Complications of Guidewires

- Plaque embolization
- Arterial dissection and perforation
- Acute closure due to vasospasm
- Subintimal wire placement
- Concertina effect (false lesion due to vasospasm produced by support wire, disappears when softer part of wire is pulled-back and placed across the so called lesions)
- Wire fracture
- Wire tip entrapment.

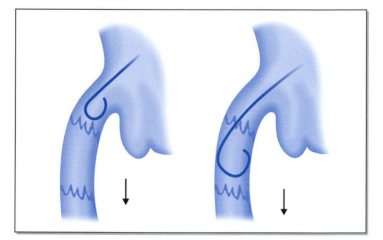

Fig. 7.15: Re-entering an already deployed stent

Suggested Reading

1. Erglis A, Narbute I, et. al. Tools and Techniques: Coronary Guidewires
2. Angled tip of the steerable guidewire and its usefulness in PTCA: Catheter Cardiovasc. Diagn : Jan Voda. 1987;13:204-10.
3. Burzotta F, Vita MD, et. al. How to solve difficult side branch access? Euro Intervention Supplement. 201;6:J72-J180.

Balloon Catheters
(The First Revolution)

■ Shuvanan Ray

Introduction

Balloon catheters are fine instruments which are manufactured with great care and engineering skill. They are often called *balloons*, and have five main parts (Fig. 8.1).

1. Balloon
2. Shaft
3. Tip
4. Central lumen for guide
5. Inflation port (inflation device).

There are mainly three types of balloons—over the wire (OTW), rapid exchange (Monorail), and fixed wire balloons. Mostly used balloons now are Monorail, where the guidewire exits a short distance about 10–30 cm back from the balloon. This allows the removal of a balloon catheter without the need to extend the guidewire and allows the operator to hold, and manipulate the guidewire and the balloon rather than relying on an assistant to secure and manipulate the guidewire as with OTW balloons.

Properties of Balloon Catheter

Entry profile: Distal tip is usually tapered, allows the balloon to cross the lesion with minimum trauma.

Crossing profile is the largest diameter in the balloon region and a low profile balloon is required to position it across tight lesions.

To cross extremely tight and long lesions both entry and crossing profiles must be low.

Most of the balloons available now do have low entry and crossing profile (Table 8.1).

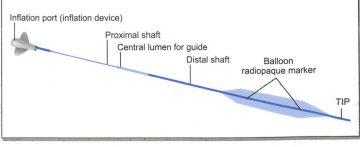

Inflation port (inflation device)
Proximal shaft
Central lumen for guide
Distal shaft
Balloon radiopaque marker
TIP

Fig. 8.1: Parts of balloon catheter

Table 8.1: Profile of different balloon catheters

Balloon	Entry profile (mm)	Crossing profile (mm)
Medtronic Sprinter 3/20 mm	0.85	1.00
Biotronik Elect 3/20 mm	0.85	1.00
Guidant Voyager 3/20 mm	0.80	0.95
Boston Scientific Maverick 3/20 mm	0.85	0.95

Inflation and Deflation Time

The balloons must be having short inflation and deflation time to avoid ischemic complication. Inflation and deflation times are the time required to transmit pressure from the indeflator to the balloon (vice versa) and the time required for the balloon material for expansion and recoil. The resistance determining inflation and deflation is the function of balloon material as well as the radius and length of the hypotube of the catheter. Low caliber catheters improve trackability of the device but low caliber catheter shaft profile leads to longer inflation and deflation time. Figure 8.2 shows the inflation and deflation times of different balloon catheters. Diminished cross-sectional area and smooth profile of the refolded balloon cause less blood flow obstruction and avoids vessel traumatization, stent damage or withdrawal.

Balloon Compliance

Change in balloon diameter for a given change in balloon pressure determines balloon compliance. According to balloon compliance, basically balloons are classified into:
- Semicompliant
- Noncompliant

Each device from each manufacturer has different compliance chart given by the manufacturer (Table 8.2).

Semicompliant balloons: They usually have moderate-to-high compliance. Usually made of either:
- Polyolefin copolymer (POC)
- Polyethylene [Less compliant than POC]

Semi-compliant balloons have a tendency of dog boning (tendency to be oversized at the edges with less dilatation at the obstructive segment of the lesion), but their crossability and trackability is superior (Fig. 8.3)

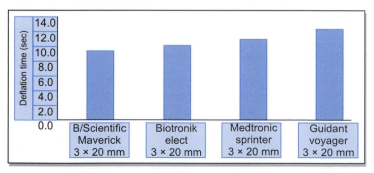

Fig. 8.2: Average deflation time to PTCA balloon catheters

Table 8.2: Compliance chart of compliant balloons

Balloon	Diameter compliance (%/bar)
Medtronic sprinter 3 x 20 mm	9.92
Biotronik elect 3 x 20 mm	5.50
Guidant voyager 3 x 20 mm	8.99
Boston Scientific Maverick 3 x 20 mm	9.88

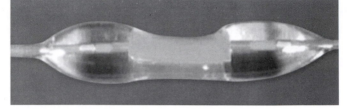

Fig. 8.3: Dog boning

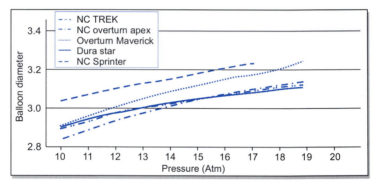

Fig. 8.4: Balloon compliance of 3 mm NC balloon catheters

Noncompliant balloons: These are basically thick-walled balloons made up of polyethylene terephthalate (PET) or nylon. They allow the operator to work at higher pressures necessary to crack hard or calcified lesion or stent postdilatation. These balloons grow very less with change of pressure. The compliance chart mostly used noncompliant balloons are given in Figure 8.4. Of the two materials, PET is more tough and generates more tensile strength and nylon balloons are softer but they rewrap better than former. So, nylon is used for balloons where rewrapping is important, e.g. cutting balloons.

Balloon Mechanics

A standard balloon is a thin-walled cylindrical pressure vessel. The stresses in a standard balloon are represented by the following equations:

Balloon will burst, if stress exceeds the rupture stress of the material.

$$\sigma_r = Pd/2t \text{ and } \sigma_l = Pd/4t$$

Where,

P = Pressure
d = Diameter
σ_r = Hoop or radial stress
σ_l = Axial or longitudinal stress
t = Thickness (as made)

From the above equation, the radial tensile strength of a balloon can be easily calculated as follows:

Ts = Calculated radial tensile strength
    = Pd/2t
Where,   P = Burst pressure
                d = Diameter (as made)
                t = Thickness (as made)

Fortunately, the radial stress or hoop stress is twice the longitudinal stress; therefore when a balloon fails it normally splits along its length rather circumferentially which is clinically desirable.

Nominal and Rated Burst Pressures

Nominal pressure is the pressure at which balloon would have expanded to the manufacturer specified size.

Rated burst pressure (RBP) is the maximum recommended pressure for safe use—99.9% of the tested balloons will not fail at RBP with 95% confidence.

The dilating force: Hoop or radial stress, which is again dependent on balloon size and compliance, is the major determinant for successful mechanical dilatation.

Cutting and Scoring Balloons

Cutting balloon angioplasty (CBA) is a technique theorized in 1980. It involves a balloon catheter equipped to incise or score the vessel lumen during angioplasty, reducing barotraumas due to high hoop stress and controlling microfissures-factors associated with neointimal hyperplasia in conventional percutaneous transluminal coronary angioplasty (PTCA). Despite the fact that CBA is seemingly optimal for ostial and fibrous lesions, randomized clinical trials did not show a very promising result. But after drug-eluting stent appearing in the scenario, CBA could be an essential tool for plaque modification before stenting, leading to better deployment and expansion of the stent (Figs 8.5 and 8.6).

Typically, cutting balloon catheters feature three or four blades or atherotomes longitudinally mounted with pad onto a balloon catheter. The mounting pad allows the atherotomes to remain fixed to the balloon. The balloon material is nylon which makes the balloon less compliant than conventional balloon catheter and are limited in traversing tortuous anatomy.

Presence of sharp blades demands slow inflation and deflation of the balloon, particularly at low pressure (<8 atm) and choosing a balloon 1 size smaller than the artery. Vessel perforation is a major risk with CBA.

Selection of Balloon Catheter

Selection of balloon catheters are less critical in stent era, but there are some general principles which need to be followed:
- Initially, a compliant balloon is selected, except in cases where rigidity/calcification is anticipated.
- Balloon to be selected according to distal arterial reference. 1:1 or a little (1 size) smaller balloon is to be selected.

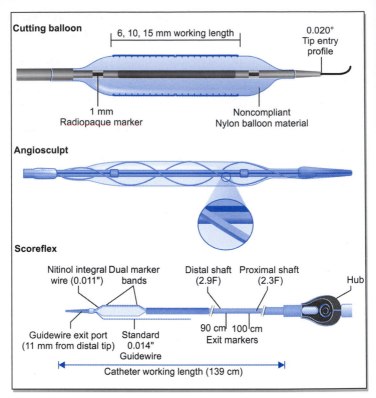

Fig. 8.5: Different scoring balloons—Cutting balloon/angiosculpt/scoreflex

Cutting balloon™ device
Lumen gain achieved primarily through plaque compression
and less to vessel wall expansion

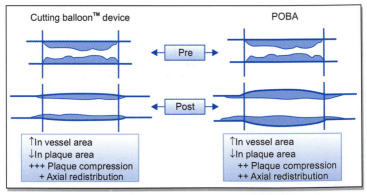

Fig. 8.6: CBA versus POBA

Abbreviations: CBA, cutting balloon angioplasty; POBA, plain old balloon angioplasty

- Balloon to be inflated at less pressure (<10 atm), if there is still a waist, then think of fibrotic or calcific lesions, requiring another device for plaque modification. Semicompliant balloons should not be inflated in very high pressure due to dog-boning effect and vessel rupture.

- In calcific or fibrotic lesion CBA or noncompliant balloons are chosen. Noncompliant balloons can be inflated to high pressure 18–20 atm to break the lesion.
- For stent postdilatation always take a short ($\leq$ 10 mm) noncompliant balloon of same size of the stent and go to high pressure. If the proximal vessel is larger, the proximal part of the stent would be dilated by higher pressure with the same balloon or a larger balloon.
- For kissing balloon inflation after stenting always take a noncompliant balloon for the side branch, which is ¼th size smaller than side branch diameter and go to high pressure for complete opening of ostium.

Drug-coated Balloons

Drug-eluting balloons (DEBs) have been developed in recent years to overcome some of the limitations of drug-eluting stent implantation, e.g. need for prolonged dual antiplatelet therapy (DAPT), and the risks of late and very late stent thrombosis.

Drug-eluting balloons are semicompliant balloons covered with antiproliferative drugs that is rapidly released upon contact with vessel wall. Expected potential benefits are avoidance of two major limitations of DES implantation.

Already, the role of DEBs are established in the treatment of bare metal or drug-eluting stent restenosis, but its role in small vessel disease (< 2.5 mm vessel and diffuse long lesion) is promising.

Facts about Drug-eluting Balloons

- Semicompliant balloon, coated with 3 µg/mm² paclitaxel, which rapidly crosses the cell membrane and binds to microtubules, inhibiting cell division, migration and proliferation of the cells.
- Coating is very important, it must prevent the drug to be washed off during transit.
- Iopromide, film-forming agent shellac, amphiphilic butyryl trihexyl citrate and urea are the most widely used coating agents (Table 8.3).
- Usually, 60 seconds is used for balloon inflation allowing a homogeneous transfer of 8–18% of the drug to the treated vessel wall (size of balloon : artery is 1.1 : 1)
- Predilatation with a smaller balloon before DEB treatment is required (0.9:1)

Table 8.3: Important drug-coated balloons

Product Name	Manufacturer	Coating	
DIOR – I	B. Braun	Iopromide	1st Generation
DIOR – II	Eurocor	Dimethyl sulfate	
ELUTAX – II	Aaachen	None	
Sequent Please	B. Braun	Iopromide	2nd generation
FALCON	Medtronic	Urea	2nd generation
MOXY	Lutonix	Polysorbate	2nd generation
PANTERA LUX	Biotronik	Butyryl trihexyl citrate	2nd generation

- Predilatation is thought to improve drug uptake by creating micro-dissections in the vessel wall, and thus facilitating drug transport through intima and media layers.
- All DEBs are not same, their drug kinetics are different, probably, their efficacy also would be different.

Suggested Reading

1. Ali R, Adam BG, Aaron D. A review of available angioplasty guiding catheters, wires and balloons. Interventional Cardiology, 2012.
2. Sigmund RA, De Mario C, Morice MC. Cutting balloon versus conventional balloon angioplasty for the treatment of in-stent restenosis (RESCUT): JACC. 2004;43(6):943.

Stents

■ Priyam Mukherjee, Shuvanan Ray

Coronary angioplasty, conceptually described by Dotter and Judkins in 1964, was first performed by Andreas Gruntzig in 1977. Coronary stents were developed in the mid-1980s and since then have seen major refinements in design and composition. The landmark events in the history of stent development are shown in Table 9.1.

WALLSTENT (Schneider AG), a self-expanding, stainless steel wire-mesh structure, was the first coronary stent implanted in a human

Table 9.1: Historical milestones in coronary artery stenting

Time	Persons(s)/Agency	Landmark events
1964	Dotter and Judkins	Conceptual description of coronary angioplasty using an implantable prosthetic device
1977	Gruntzig and Myler	First coronary angioplasty during coronary artery bypass graft surgery
1977	Andreas Gruntzig	First coronary angioplasty in an awake patient; a revolution in interventional cardiology
1979	Geoffrey Hartzler	First balloon angioplasty to treat AMI
1986	Sigwart and Puel	The first implantation of a stent in human coronary arteries; second revolution in intervention cardiology
1991	Cannon and Roubin	First coronary stenting to treat AMI
1994	Serruys et al. and Fischman et al.	Publication of first two landmark (Benestent and STRESS) trials
1994	FDA	FDA-approved use of stents to treat acute and threatened vessel closure after failed balloon angioplasty
1999	Eduardo Sousa	The first drug (sirolimus) eluting stent implanted in human coronary artery; third revolution in interventional cardiology
2002–04	EMA and FDA	Approvals of Cypher and Taxus stents in Europe and USA
2011	EMA	Approval of Absorb BVS (bioresorbable vascular scaffold) in Europe; fourth revolution in interventional cardiology

Abbreviations: FDA, Food and Drug Administration; EMA, European Medicines Agency; AMI, acute myocardial infarction.

coronary artery by Sigwart et al. in 1986. The technical challenges in using the stent delivery system (an inner shaft and outer constraining sheath) limited its clinical utility and it was withdrawn from market in 1991. Schatz and co-workers developed the Palmaz-Schatz (Johnson & Johnson) stent in 1987, the first FDA-approved stent in the USA. It was the first balloon-expandable, stainless steel, slotted tube device and remained one of the most studied and widely used stent in 1990s. Many other stents were subsequently developed in early 1990s and included: Flexstent (Cook), Wiktor (Medtronic), Micro (Applied Vascular Engineering), Cordis (Cordis) and Multi-link (Advanced Cardiovascular Systems). The use of these stents, indeed, reduced early elastic recoil and restenosis seen with plain old balloon angioplasty (POBA). However, this new technology was not without its drawbacks. These initial stents had high metallic density, resulting in a high incidence of subacute stent thrombosis (ST), and were bulky and technically challenging to use, resulting in frequent failure in deployment and embolization. Furthermore, these initial coronary stents, although reduced the incidence of restenosis compared with POBA, were still at a significant risk of in-stent restenosis (ISR). These technical challenges and potential complications kept the use of stents limited to the cases of acute or threatened closure or restenosis after POBA. In 1993, two landmark trials, the Belgium Netherlands Stent Arterial Revascularization Therapies Study (BENESTENT) and the North American Stent Restenosis Study (STRESS), demonstrated superiority of the bare metal stents (BMS) over POBA, thus establishing coronary stent implantation as an accepted standard of care for percutaneous coronary intervention (PCI). The use of coronary stents increased exponentially over the next few years and by 1999, stents were used in nearly 85% of PCI procedures. However, the medium and longer term follow-up of BMS revealed as high as 20–30% incidence of in-stent restenosis (ISR), due to proliferation and migration of vascular smooth muscle cells (VSMCs) within the stents. ISR may be associated with significant morbidity and mortality and the drug-eluting stents (DES) were developed to specifically address the problems of ISR encountered with BMS.

The TAXUS Express and Cypher (Cordis, Miami Lakes, FL, USA) DES are examples of first generation platforms that established the foundation for the development of newer-generation DES. The TAXUS paclitaxel-eluting stent (PES) consisted of a SS (stainless steel) scaffold with a 132 μm strut plus 22 μm polymer thickness, whereas the Cypher sirolimus-eluting stent (SES) consisted of a SS scaffold of 140 μm strut thickness with a 13 μm polymer layer. These first-generation stents served as main comparators to contemporary DES in multiple clinical trials. The TAXUS Liberte is a PES on a SS hybrid design scaffold with a strut thickness of 97 μm with a 16 μm thick layer of triblock polymer matrix of polystyrene-b-isobutylene-b-styrene) and a paclitaxel concentration of 10 pg/mm^2 with very slow drug-release kinetics, leading to less than 10% paclitaxel elution during the initial 28 days. The TAXUS Element PES (ION stent) is a next-generation system with the same polymer and drug components on a Pt-Cr open cell design scaffold of 81 μm strut thickness (Element scaffold design) that was approved by the FDA in 2011. Platinum chromium ensures more visibility of the stents.

The Endeavor (Medtronic, Minneapolis, MN, USA) platform is a zotarolimus-eluting stents (ZES) consisting of a Co-Cr open cell scaffold of 91 μm strut thickness and a 6 μm polymer layer thickness. It contains a zotarolimus concentration of 10 μg/mm stent length (or 160 g/cm²) and a highly biocompatible hydrophilic phosphorylcholine polymer that results in very rapid drug-elution profile, with greater than 95% eluted in the initial 14 days postimplantation. Very early resolution of drug increases the chance of neointimal proliferation as a result more stent-related hazards. The Endeavor Resolute ZES (Medtronic, Minneapolis, MN, USA) has endeavor platform and drug concentration as the Endeavor ZES (E-ZEES) but contains a BioLinx polymer that is highly biocompatible and provides slower release kinetics with 85%, of drug eluted over 2 months and complete elution by 6 months. The Integrity BMS is a new iteration of the Driver TM BMS (Medtronic, Inc., Santa Rosa, CA, USA); the zotarolimus-eluting version is the Resolute integrity stent where integrity BMS replaces the driver platform in the new stent. The integrity stent platform uses a single cobalt chromium wire to form a continuous sinusoidal pattern of crowns and struts wrapped helically around a mandrel with a 0.09 mm strut thickness and a 1.12 mm crossing profile. This unique manufacturing technology enhances stent flexibility, deliverability, and conformability without sacrificing radial strength. Bench test confirmed that the Resolute integrity DES was more resistant to longitudinal distortion in elongation tests than the Omega element or driver stents, and similar to the other stents tested. The resolute integrity and the driver platform have two connections compared with three for Xience V and Xience Prime stents results in more flexibility at the same time the unique helical single-wire design decreases the longitudinal distortion of the Resolute and integrity stent, thus, maintaining a balance between flexibility and longitudinal integrity.

The next generation Resolute stent, Resolute Onyx™ is composed of a composite wire material consisting of a platinum iridium alloy core, resulting in improved radiopacity as compared with Resolute Integrity™ ZES (RI-ZES, Medtronic, Inc.), and a shell composed of the same cobalt alloy material as RI-ZES. Utilization of this novel, core wire technology enables the Resolute Onyx ZES to improve radiopacity, despite being composed of thinner stent struts as compared with Resolute Integrity ZES (81 μm vs 91 μm, respectively). These changes result in a lower crossing profile (1.04 mm vs 1.12 mm) and facilitate improved tracking and lesion crossing. Resolute Onyx ZES showed to be 20% more trackable than RI-ZES based on a lower mean maximum force required to pass through a simulated tortuosity model. To negate any compromise in radial strength, the Resolute Onyx ZES adopts an increased strut width to thickness ratio. It has sizes starting from 2.0 mm to 4.5 and 5.0 mm. It has same continuous sinusoidal technology (CST) as integrity.

Everolimus-eluting Stents

XIENCE V—the cobalt chromium EES has a strut thickness of 81 μg and is coated with a 7.6 μg thick nonerodible copolymer of polyvinylidene fluoride co-hexafluoropropylene and poly-n-butyl methacrylate which facilitates the elution of Everolimus over 120 days.

Numerous randomized studies have compared the performance of EES with BMS, SES, PES and ZES. More recently the XIENCE stent has also been compared with the platinum chromium PROMUS stent platform.

XIENCE PRIME—this represents the next generation EES from ABBOTT Vascular, Santa Clara, CA, USA. This has a new enhanced stent delivery system, enabling the stent to be more flexible and deliverable, with longer stent lengths being available compared to the older generation XIENCE V. The balloon also has a higher rated burst pressure at 18 atmospheres compared to 16 atmospheres with a previous generation XIENCE V. The efficacy of this stent was studied in the SPIRIT PRIME study.

XIENCE XPEDITION is the latest generation of the XIENCE family of stents. It has enhanced deliverability with change in the balloon design to ensure rapid deflation. It is available in 48 mm in length.

The Promus Premier (Boston Scientific,. Natick,, MA, USA) is a Pt-Cr EES 81 µm strut thickness and 8 µm polymer thickness on an Element open cell stent platform. The polymer, drug concentration and elution characteristics are otherwise the same as the Xience Alpine Co-Cr EES.

Device-related Safety Outcomes: Insights from Mechanical and Device Integrity and Failure

Stent Fracture

The safety of contemporary DES platforms can be evaluated from 2 distinct perspectives: (1) a device-centric model, centered on the risk of adverse events secondary to type of drug released or to mechanical device failure as determined by stent strut fracture and stent longitudinal deformation; and (2) a clinical standpoint, centered on the risk of ST and risk for target lesion revascularization (TLR). Certain device specific characteristics have been associated with adverse clinical events. For example, certain risk factors have been recognized to increase the risk of strut fracture, which in turn has been shown to be related to higher rates of clinically evident restenosis, aneurysm formation, myocardial infarction (MI), and TLR. Some of the recognized risk factors for stent fracture include lesion complexity (e.g. length, degree of calcification, vessel tortuosity, and angulation), deployment characteristic (overlapping stents, higher inflation pressure), and anatomic location (hinge points, right coronary artery, or ostial implantation). Current research is ongoing in further understanding the causes, mechanisms, and underlying microenvironment stresses and strains driving this phenomenon and associated complications. Stent fracture is an uncommon complication, with a historical incidence ranging between 0.9% and 13.4%, with a 4.0% incidence on recent meta-analysis of over 5000 subjects. Importantly, however, first-generation DES platforms with a SS closed-cell stent design and sirolimus elution were included and represented approximately 90% of the reported cases, while the remaining 10% were evenly distributed among all the contemporary platforms. A separate registry analysis of over 9000 subjects reported a strut fracture incidence rate of 1.25% in contemporary platforms. Improvement in stent design, with reduction of the number of connectors between rings from 6 S-connectors (first generation DES, leading to decreased flexibility, stiffer stent frame) to 2–3 connectors in contemporary DES designs, have been largely responsible for these observations of decreased fracture despite decreasing strut thickness.

Longitudinal Deformation

Longitudinal deformation has been discussed as another potential mechanical complication of novel stent platforms, particularly given the shift toward open cell designs to allow for improved trackability while maintaining radial strength. These designs have decreased number of interconnectors between the stent rings and have been a perceived higher risk of longitudinal stent deformation or pseudofracture, which appears most commonly in the element platform design with its distinct offset peak-to-peak interconnected ring design. Although clinical outcomes with Pt-Cr EES element stent design has decreased longitudinal strength, making it potentially vulnerable to longitudinal shortening. To prevent this complication the next generation promus stent that is, promus premier has extraconnector at its edges. Limited data are available regarding the incidence and associated clinical outcomes from longitudinal stent deformation but, in limited series, it occurs in 0.1–1.0% of contemporary DES platforms. It seems to be related to stent design characteristics, with a higher incidence for the offset peak-to-peak design (Promus Element platform) observed both clinically in limited, retrospective analyses and in in vitro engineering longitudinal compression models. Of note and as expected, longitudinal Promus Element are similar to other second-generation DES, bench studies suggest the Promus deformation was rarely observed with the stiffer early-generation DES platforms. Despite reports of increased risk of longitudinal deformation with novel thin strut stents and potential association to stent thrombosis (ST) it seems to be a rare occurrence that is mostly related to attempts to pass equipment through secondary devices during PCI.

Pathologic Correlates of Stent Fracture

Pathologic and autopsy studies have shed additional light into the clinical significance of this problem. Although historical incidence was reported at 1–2%, autopsy studies have reported a higher incidence. However, only the most severe types of stent fractures causing gaps in stented segments were associated with adverse histologic findings on pathologic studies. Contemporary Co--Cr EES platforms also seem to have decreased risk of strut fracture despite the thinner strut profiles compared with PES or SES and improved strut coverage with less evidence of inflammation, fibrin deposition, and late and very late ST (VLST). Despite these pathologic findings, fracture-related restenosis or thrombosis was comparable.

Patient-related Safety Outcomes

Insights from clinical experience from a clinical perspective, and as previously discussed, first-generation DES platforms markedly decreased the risk of restenosis and have led to improved clinical outcomes. The safety of first generation and contemporary DES platforms has centered mostly on the risk of ST. It represents a rare but potentially serious complication with a high morbidity and mortality. First-generation DES platforms were found to have similar rates of early (0–30 days) and late (31–360 days) ST compared with the BMS. However, safety concerns arose with reports of significantly increased, and persistent, annual risk of very late ST (VLST) of approximately 0.5% for up to 5 years postimplantation compared with BMS.

Pathologic studies shed insight these complications because late ST and VLST seem to have distinct mechanisms between SES and PETS platforms. Interestingly, SES specimens showed evidence of a hypersensitivity reaction with diffuse extensive inflammation, whereas PES specimens showed late stent malapposition with excessive fibrin deposition. Second-generation DES, with their improvements in scaffold design, polymer biocompatibility, and antiproliferative drug content, concentration, and elution kinetics, have significantly decreased this risk by addressing these failure mechanisms: pathologic studies of contemporary EES platforms have been shown to result in improved strut coverage and endothelialization, resulting in a decreased inflammatory response, less fibrin deposition, and decreased evidence of late and VLST compared with first generation SES and PETS in human autopsy analysis.

A large network meta-analysis of 52,158 subjects enrolled in 51 trials with follow-up of at least 3 years, compared the long-term safety of DES to BMS up to a mean of 3.8 years, and found improved efficacy and safety profile of DES with lower rates of definite ST and target vessel revascularization (TVR), with improved efficacy of Co-C:r EES compared with earlier generation DES platforms. Of note, although the EXAMINATION (A Clinical Evaluation of Everolimus Eluting Coronary Stents in the Treatment of Patients With ST-segment Elevation Myocardial Infarction) trial did not demonstrate superiority of Co-Cr EES to BMS with respect to subject-oriented endpoints in the ST- segment elevation MI (STEMI) population at 1-year follow-up, 5-year follow-up data demonstrated lower rates of these endpoints, including all-cause mortality. Importantly, TILR and ST rates were consistently lower with DES. In addition to meta-analyses, data from a recent large, randomized study of dual antiplatelet therapy duration has shed additional light into the safety of contemporary DES platforms. A prospective, propensity-matched analysis of subjects enrolled in the dual antiplatelet therapy (DAPT) study comparing 12   and30months of dual antiplatelet in 10,026 subjects (8308 with DES vs 1718 with BMS;) showed a lower risk of ST with DES compared with BMS (1.7% vs 2.6%, P = .01).

EES versus PES

Five randomized trials have compared the two with increasingly complex lesions. Irrespective of patients or lesion subsets, the EES performs better than the PES in all the trials. Consistent with these are the results of EXECUTIVE trial, which enrolled multivessel disease patients. This reported in-stent late lumen loss at 9 months follow-up of 0.08 mm (95% CI- 0.01,0.15) and 0.22 mm (95% CI- 0.13,0.31). p-value of 0.018 among patients randomized to EES and PES respectively. Longer angiographic follow-up study is available in the SPIRIT II trial, with evidence of late catch up in late lumen loss in the EES group, such that the in-stent late loss between EES and PES observed at 6 months is no longer present at 2 years. Nevertheless, the clinical outcomes at 3 years and 4 years follow-up in the SPIRIT II study remain consistent with those seen at 6 months and 1 year. Similarly in the SPIRIT III trial at

5 years follow-up, the EES has significantly lower rates of MACE. More extensive assessments of EES took place in the SPIRIT IV trial and the all comers COMPARE trial. At 3 years follow-up both studies reported superior efficacy and safety with EES compared to PES. Furthermore, the SPIRIT IV and COMPARE trials were the first to report lower stent thrombosis in the EES group compared to PES group.

EES versus SES

Several studies have compared the EES with the SES, which is the most efficacious first generation DES. The EXCELLENT trial randomized 3:1 EES to SES, the study achieved its prespecified noninferiority primary end point of in segment late lumen loss at 9 months. At 12 months follow-up there was no significant difference in the rates of MACE, myocardial infarction, TLR with lower stent thrombosis in the EES group. At 3 years follow-up, both the efficacy and safety remained numerically better with EES compared to SES.

Biodegradable Polymers

Supportive backbones, polymer coatings or carriers and antirestenotic drugs contribute to the efficacy and safety of drug-eluting stents (DES). In particular, the combination of polymer carriers with active drugs (the so-called 'matrix') has a main role in the performance of a DES. A polymer coating should ideally regulate drug-release kinetics without further interaction with the vasculature. In contrast, some polymer coatings persist in the implanted vessel wall long after their useful function has been served. These nonerodable or durable polymers may elicit a chronic inflammatory response at the site of stent implantation with possible neoatherosclerosis and stent thrombosis (ST) over the long-term.

Biodegradable-polymer DES are regarded as alternative to durable-polymer DES. Indeed, once the active drug is eluted and the polymer-coating degraded, the remaining stent backbone resembles that of a bare metal stent. In virtue of the biodegradable nature of the polymer coating, the ambitious goal of this technology is to reduce the risk for ST and the need for prolonged antiplatelet therapy compared with earlier DES platforms. Clinical investigations displayed that in comparison with early generation DES, those stents eluting antirestenotic drugs from a biodegradable polymer have superior long-term safety and efficacy. In contrast, the potential advantages of these platforms versus new-generation durable-polymer DES appear less obvious.

The followings are the currently available DES with biodegradable polymers:

BIOMATRIX Stent (Biosensors International Pvt Ltd, Singapore)

This stent elutes Biolimus A9. This was compared with the SES in an all comers population. It was found to be noninferior to SES for the primary composite endpoint of death, MI and TVR. However, after 1 year, the rate of stent thrombosis was found to be significantly lower for the Biomatrix stent.

NOBORI Stent (Terumo, Japan)

This stent utilizes the same PLA polymer and the antiproliferative agent as Biomatrix, however, the Nobori uses the S stent platform, while the Biomatrix stent uses the Juno stent platform. The Nobori has been compared with the Cypher and the Taxus stents. In the nonrandomized NOBORI CORE study, the reported late loss at 9 months was similar between the two groups, but the restoration of endothelial function was better with the Nobori Stent. In the NOBORI 1 study the stent was compared with the Taxus stent, and the stent was found to have better outcomes compared with Taxus, in terms of late loss. Similarly the rates of stent thrombosis were lower in the Nobori group. The NOBORI is now being compared with the XIENCE stent in the COMPARE 2 trial.

Synergy Stent (Boston Scientific)

New generation biodegradable polymer containing stent Synergy has definite advantage regarding continuation of DAPT. Synergy contains thin-strut (74–81 µm), PtCr metal alloy platform with an ultrathin (4 µmol/L) bioabsorbable Poly (D,L lactide-co-glycolide) abluminal polymer, which elutes everolimus (100 µg/cm²). Polymer of the stent degrades at around three months. In a patient where there is a higher risk of bleeding this stent can be helpful due to provision of early DAPT discontinuation.

Polymer-free Stents

Here the aim was to remove the polymer altogether as polymer could be the cause of adverse events. The advantages of a polymer-free DES includes rapid healing, an improvement in the integrity of the stent's surface owing to the absence of a polymer cracking or peeling-off or webbing of the polymer. Several techniques are available to permit drug elution from a polymer-free stent.

1. The bioactive substance can directly be attached to the stent surface by covalent bonding.
2. The bioactive substance can be dissolved in a nonpolymeric biodegradable carrier on the stent surface.
3. The bioactive agent in its pure form can be impregnated into the porous surface of the stent or into the stent's body

YUKON–Sirolimus-eluting Stent

This is a stainless steel stent and is the first polymer-free stent studied. The stent has a microporous surface with pores, which are 2 µg deep. And functions as a reservoir for the drug. The dose of the Sirolimus can be customized in the Cathlab before implantation, in a coating process that takes around 8 minutes. After complete drug release, the microporous surface facilitates the adhesion of endothelial cells. A process confirmed by OCT Randomized data include no inferiority compared with PES. The ISAR TEST compared Yukon with the PES, showing comparable TLR, death or MI. Observational studies have suggested that in the long-term Yukon may have lower rates of delayed restenosis compared with Sirolimus-eluting durable polymer stents. A lower significant change in late loss between 6 months to 2 years for the Yukon stent was observed compared with the durable polymer based Sirolimus-eluting stents.

BIOFREEDOM Biolimus A9-eluting Stent

This is a polymer-free Biolimus-eluting stent, made of stainless steel, with a strut thickness of 112 µg, and a microstructured polymer-free surface alteration. More than 90% of the drug is released in around 50 hours. This has been compared to the Taxus Liberte Stent in a randomized trial, with the primary endpoint of late loss at 4 months. Late loss at 4 months was significantly lower compared with the Taxus stent. This angiographic finding was confirmed by intravascular ultrasound (IVUS).

Tapered Stents

Meril Life Science has introduced long tapered stent Biomime Morph for long diffuse disease. The distal diameter of the stent is 0.5 mm less than the proximal diameter (2.75/2.25,3.0/2.5, 3.5/3.0). The length available in the market is 30 mm, 40 mm, 50 mm and 60 mm. It is a sirolimus-eluting stent with ultrathin sturt of 65 µm. It has a hybrid design with closed cell design at both ends which prevents it from longitudinal shortening. Rest of the stent has an open cell design for better side branch access. Though long-term data is lacking for the stent.

Bioresorbable Vascular Scaffolds

The limitations of balloon angioplasty were serious flow limiting dissections and acute recoil leading to abrupt closure. This problem was overcome with the introduction of BMS, which provided a mechanical scaffold. However, this lead to significant vessel wall injury, much more than plain balloon angioplasty, and leading to restenosis resulting from neointimal hyperplasia. This problem of neointimal hyperplasia leading to restenosis was addressed by the DES, which lead to significantly lower restenosis rates. However, the persistence of the polymer lead to late problems like very late stent thrombosis, late acquired stent malapposition and neoatherosclerosis. Fully bioresorbable DES have been specifically designed to overcome these problems.

Absorbable Metal Stent Biotronik (Biotronik, Berlin, Germany) manufactured a balloon expandable Absorbable Metallic Stent (AMS), composed of the magnesium alloy. The first generation stent was investigated in the progress AMS trial, but the results were disappointing with a very high TLR (45%), at 1 year. A newer generation of the scaffold AMS 3 DREAMS (Drug Eluting AMS) with slow degeneration time and with Paclitaxel elution has been evaluated in the BIOSOLVE 1 study. Results have been promising with, with a target lesion failure, and clinically driven TLR of 10% at two years. DREAMS has been modified to DREAMS 2, which possesses tantalum radiopaque end markers, and elutes Sirolimus. The FIM study to assess DREAMS 2, BIOSOLVE II, will be recruiting patients in the future.

The more promising concept is the fully Biodegradable BVS, introduced by Abbott Vascular (Santa Clara, CA, USA). It contains the crystalline poly (L lactide) backbone on top of which Everolimus is applied in the form of poly D-L lactide acid. This has been investigated in the FIM ABSORB cohort A and B, with promising results. The ABSORB Extend included more complex lesions, with a 1 year ischemia driven TLR of 2%, and stent thrombosis of 0.8%. Long-term follow-up of Absorb BVS is not very much encouraging.

Conclusion

First generation stents Cypher (SES) and Taxus (PES) have their own drawbacks. Pathological studies have clearly shown that Cypher stent causes chronic vascular inflammation even after one year leading to late and very late stent thrombosis. On the other hand PES causes positive vascular remodeling leading to late stent malapposition and fibrin deposition and hence predisposd to late and very late stent thrombosis. The old generation polymer is responsible for the chronic inflammation and the drug paclitaxel has its own demerit that it remains in the vessel for long duration leading to incomplete endothelialization. These factors are responsible for neoatherosclerosis which may lead to very late stent thrombosis. Pathological studies have shown that the incidence of neoatherosclerosis is higher in DES over two years than BMS. So the challenge was to combat these issues and with newer modifications second generation stents came in the market. There was evolution of stent in terms of strut thickness, platform composition and design and last but not the least the new generation polymer. Regarding the antiproliferative drug Medtronic introduced Endeavor sprint which has zotarolimus as new drug. But the stents did not achieve good reputation in the market due to its higher events rates. This was due to very fast drug release kinetics . An ideal stent should have optimum drug concentration and release kinetic such that the drug should be in the lumen for at least three months and should not be more than six months. The logic behind these type of kinetics that it should prevent neointimal proliferation in early phase of stent deployment and at the same time should not prevent endothelialization of the stent strut in long run otherwise one has to continue DAPT for long duration to prevent stent thrombosis.

Polymer is an important issue regarding stent quality. First generation stents have been condemned for their polymer quality. The second generation stents have more biocompatible polymes like fluoropolymer which cause less vascular inflammation and hence less incidence of stent thrombosis compared to first generation DES. But still pathological studies have shown that the incidence of neoatherosclerosis is as high as first generation DES. Thus, there is always chance of late and very late stent thrombosis even with newer biocompatible polymers. So an ideal stent should have either no polymer or biodegradable polymer. Stents with biodegradable polymer will behave as BMS once the drug elution has been completed and after polymer degradation took place. It has been clearly demonstrated that BMS has less neoatherosclerosis compared to DES at two years and even after six years. DAPT can be stopped earlier in these stents.

Regarding stent design, an ideal stent should have thin strut so that their will be less metal burden. Metal burden is related to stent thrombosis. Newer generation stents have thinner struts, they are more trackable and flexible, can take the shape of vessel so less shear force on the stent and less chance of late stent fracture.

In osteal location or left main stenting one should not choose stents which are notorious for longitudinal shortening. In tortuous vessel one should opt for more trackable stents like Resolute integrity, Resolute Onyx or Synergy. Open cell design are better than closed or semiclosed design stents in doing bifurcation stenting for better side branch access. Bioabsorbable scaffold though looks good but lacks long-term superior results and should be used judiciously. One has to continue DAPT for prolong duration and BVS implantation should be avoided in complex lesion like calcified vessel or osteal location.

Suggested Reading

1. Foerst J, Vorpahl M, Engelhardt M, et al. Evolution of coronary stents: from bare-metal stent so fully biodegradable, drug-eluting stents. Comb Prod Ther. 2013;3:9-24.
2. Iqbal A, Gunn J, Serruys PW. Coronary stents: historical development, current status and future directions. British Medical Bulletin. 2013;106:193-211.
3. Lee SWL, Chan MPH, Chan KKW. Acute and 16-month outcomes of a new stent: the first-in-man evaluation of the medtronic S9 (Integrity) stent: Catheterization and Cardiovascular Interventions. 2011;78:898-908.
4. Simard T, Hibbert B, Ramirez D, et al. The evolution of coronary stents: a brief review. Canadian Journal of Cardiology. 2014;30:35-45.
5. Yahagi K, Joner M, Virmani R. Insights into very late stent thrombosis from the wisdom of pathology. The Journal of Invasive Cardiology. 2014;26(9):417-9.

Nonangiographic Lesion Assessment
(Adjunct Devices)

■ Shuvanan Ray

Coronary angiography is basically a luminogram and cannot see the structures beyond the ceiling. Moreover, the lesion assessment in a bent or curved artery or in eccentric location can make the assessment by angiography sometimes difficult. Adjunct devices help the clinician to assess whether the lesion is anatomically or hemodynamically significant to develop ischemia. Adjunct devices are used to delineate either the anatomy of the lesion or to assess its physiological significance.

Anatomical assessment can be augmented by using intravascular ultrasound (IVUS) and optical coherence tomography (OCT), whereas physiological assessment is done by using fractional flow reserve (FFR) and instantaneous wave-free flow ratio (IFR) which gives an estimate of hemodynamic significance of the lesion.

Fractional Flow Reserve

Fractional flow reserve (FFR) is measured as the ratio of mean distal coronary pressure divided by mean proximal aortic pressure during maximal hyperemia. The coronary pressure beyond the stenosis is measured with a 0.014 inch guide wire with high fidelity pressure transducer mounted 3 cm from the tip of the wire at the junction of radiopaque and radiolucent segments.

FFR is defined as the ratio of maximal hyperemic flow across an epicardial artery with stenosis compared with maximal hyperemic flow in the same artery without stenosis.

It is seen that coronary angiography can detect only 5% of coronary tree but 95% of the distribution remains beyond angiographic assessment and it constitutes the microcirculation which almost reach each myocardial fiber. The larger epicardial arteries are called conductance vessels and smaller arteries called resistance arteries because collectively they setup the tone of microcirculation to increase blood flow when necessary. During exercise, there is vasodilatation of both conductance and resistance to produce increased blood flow (3–4 times than normal). When there is a stenosis in the epicardial artery, the microcirculation dilates to increase the circulation with limited supply (Fig. 10.1).

FFR depends on a principle that there will be no difference in mean pressure between aorta and distal coronary bed during maximal hyperemia, if there is no stenosis of the supplying artery.

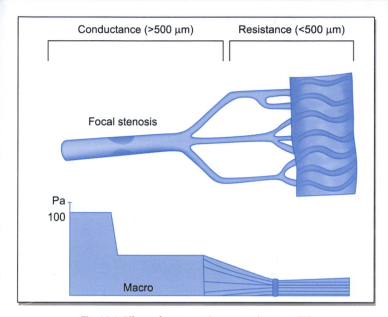

Fig. 10.1: Effects of macro- and microcirculation on FFR

$$FFR = Pd/Pa = 1$$

Pd = mean distal coronary pressure at maximal hyperemia/Pa = mean aortic P at maximal hyperemia

If FFR is 0.6, then it means that due to the particular stenosis in the epicardial artery, maximum achievable blood flow to the myocardium by this artery is only 60% of what it would be if this coronary artery were completely normal.

FFR also accounts for the following factors:
1. Size of the perfusion area (Fig. 10.2).
2. Collateral circulation (Fig. 10.3).
3. Microvascular dysfunction (impaired microcirculation).

* Fractional flow reserve (FFR) may be false negative in presence of microvascular dysfunction (ST elevation myocardial infarction) and severe LV hypertrophy.

* FFR may be over-estimated, if caffeine/methyl xanthine is used concurrently.

Technique of Fractional Flow Reserve

FFR can be easily measured using a 5F or 6F guide catheter and either of two available pressure wire systems (St Jude Medical, Minneapolis or Volcano Therapeutics, Rancho, Cordova, CA). After diagnostic angiography with catheter seated in coronary ostium, the following steps are necessary:
1. Femoral venous sheath (necessary for central IV infusion of adenosine).
2. The pressure wire is connected to the system's pressure analyzer and calibrated and zeroed outside body.
3. Intracoronary nitroglycerine (100–200 µg) bolus given.

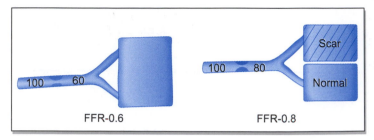

Fig. 10.2: FFR and size of perfusion area

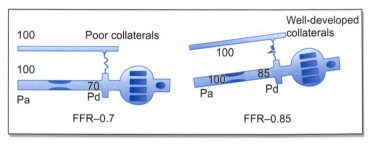

Fig. 10.3: FFR and collated circulation

4. The wire is advanced through the guide to the coronary artery. The pressure wire signal and the guide pressure are matched before crossing the stenosis.
5. The wire is then advanced across the stenosis about 2 cm distal to the coronary artery.
6. Maximal hyperemia is induced with IV adenosine (140 µg/kg/min) × 2 minutes (via central vein)/IC adenosine [20–30 µg for RCA and 60–100 µg for LCA] (Tables 10.1 and 10.2).
7. FFR is calculated.

IC Adenosine versus IV Adenosine for Fractional Flow Reserve

- IV adenosine is the standard procedure for induction of maximal coronary hyperemia (Table 10.1).
  – Expensive
  – Needs IV access
  – Allows pull back.
  (Particularly helpful in tandem, diffuse lesions)
- IC adenosine is an acceptable alternative (Table 10.2), cheaper does not require venous access, but does not allow pull back and does not produce steady state maximal hyperemia
  15 ampoules of adenosine (Sanofi) = 15 × 2 mL = 30 mL = 90 mg
  Add with 60 mL of NS = 90 mg in 90 mL = 1 mg/mL.

Clinical Use of Fractional Flow Reserve

- *Left main stenosis:* Intermediate lesions in LMCA can be assessed by FFR and treatment strategy is planned. FFR-negative cases can be

Table 10.1: Preparation of IV adenosine

Adenosine IV infusion		
1 mg/mL		
Weight (kg)	140 µg/kg/min = 8.4 mg/kg/hour Infusion rate (mL/hr)	180 µg/kg/min = 10.8 mg/kg/hour Infusion rate (mL/hr)
45	378	486
50	420	540
55	462	594
60	504	648
65	546	702
70	588	756
75	630	810
80	672	864
85	714	918
90	756	972
95	798	1026
100	840	1080
115	882	1188
120	924	1242
125	1050	1296

Table 10.2: Preparation of IC adenosine

IC adenosine
1 amp = 6 mg = 2 mL + 4 mL NS   = 1 mg/mL + 99 mL of NS = 10 µg/mL
RCA = 40 µg
LCA = 60 µg
Increase to max 150 µg, if FFR is 0.75–0.85

treated medically, and there is no difference in mortality between surgical and nonsurgical cases.

- *Multivessel disease:* FFR in multi-vessel CAD can reduce the number of stents and lower cost. FAME study demonstrated that PCI-guided by FFR significantly reduced mortality and myocardial infarction at 2 years compared with angiography guided PCI.
- *Ostial and side branch lesions:* Measurement of FFR for ostial and side branch assessment identifies the minority of lesions that are functionally significant, reducing the need for complex time consuming and potentially detrimental side branch intervention.
- *Diffuse or tandem lesion:* If the lesions are situated at a distance more than 6 times the vessel diameter, they behave independently. In clinical practice, use of pressure pull-back recording is helpful to identify the effect of individual stenosis. Continuous and gradual pressure recovery from distal to proximal, during pull-back characterizes a diffuse lesion. If there is a abrupt change in any focal region that area demands treatment as an appropriate location.

Instantaneous Wave-free Ratio (IFR)

Instantaneous wave-free ratio (IFR) is performed using high fidelity pressure wire across the lesion. IFR isolates a specific period in diastole, called wave-free period, and uses the ratio of distal coronary pressure (Pd) to the pressure observed in aorta (Pa) over this period. When stenosis is flow limiting, Pd and Pa over the wave-free period diverge and IFR values become < 0.90 (in place of 1 in normal) which suggests flow limitation. It is measured at rest, without the need of pharmacological vasodilators.

Different studies [ADVICE, CLARIFY], confirm that IFR and FFR values are correlated with the classification of the coronary stenosis severity, indicating that IFR can be used as an adenosine-free alternative to FFR.

Intravascular Imaging (IVUS, OCT)

As it is known that coronary angiogram is a luminogram in 2D format, interventional community needed something to see beyond that. From angiography it appears that atherosclerotic process is focal but autopsy studies, consistently demonstrate that atherosclerotic process is actually diffuse. So, the focal lesions as detected buy angiography are more diseased and mildly "irregular" segments are almost always diseased as well.

Arterial remodeling is another phenomenon which is often missed by angiography. It is seen that with increasing plaque volume the arterial wall is also displaced outward. This compensatory enlargement allows the artery to accommodate a certain amount of plaque volume without affecting the lumen. Stenosis of lumen takes place when this compensatory mechanism fails, i.e. plaque volume becomes more in comparison to enlargement.

So, remodeled arterial segment with significant plaque burden may be angiographically normal. Again, luminal narrowing may take place more in comparison to plaque volume, which is called negative remodeling and it is actually due to reduction in the size of the artery itself. It is said that positive remodeling is found mostly in acute coronary syndrome and negative remodeling in stable ischemic heart disease. (Fig. 10.4).

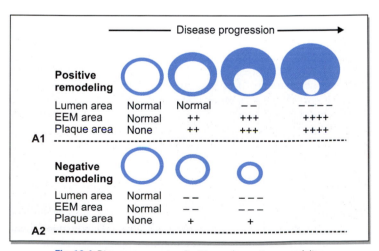

Fig. 10.4: Disease progression: Positive and negative remodeling

Also the complexity of the lesions make angiography look inadequate in planning and performing PCI, in certain situations like ostial lesions, bifurcation lesions, calcified lesions, unprotected left main artery disease, where more clarification of image is required. Particularly, more so, in the present era where, every day more and more challenging cases are coming for PCI.

Intravascular Ultrasound

Two types of intravascular ultrasound (IVUS) systems are available:
1. A mechanical system that relies on rotational internal cable.
2. A solid state system, mounted on a catheter and electronically controlled.

In the mechanical system, the imaging core rotates via a flexible drive shaft through a 360° arc in the vessel, generating 30 images per second.

The solid state catheter has 64 ultrasound transducers arranged circumferentially around the catheter tip and sequentially activated to produce a 360° image.

Both catheters are 6F compatible.

Image features (Fig. 10.5) are described from center to periphery:
1. *Dead zone:* The black circular ring in the middle of the image is caused by space occupied by the catheter.
2. *Catheter artefacts:* This is a halo artefact around the catheter (may be due to imaging sheath or disorganized near-field echo signals—ring down).
3. *Lumen:* The dark echolucent area surrounding the catheter artefact signal is the lumen.
4. *Inner layer:* In a normal artery, intima is difficult to detect. The thin inner echogenic layer surrounding the lumen, usually represent the internal elastic lamina.
5. Middle hypoechoic layer is the media.
6. Outer echogenic layer is adventitia.

Intimal thickening is the hallmark of arterial wall disease. When the intima thickness becomes more echodense and easier to visualize on display. The echodense intimal leading edge defines the boundaries of the lumen, while the leading edge of the adventitia, the external

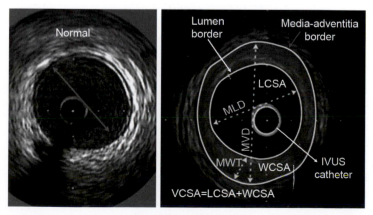

Fig. 10.5: Image features

elastic lamina defines the vessel area. The area between both tracings is considered as plaque plus media, or atheroma area.

IVUS Measurement in Practice

There are two important interfaces in an IVUS image – the lumen-intima and media-adventitia interfaces. They are generally accurate through means of ultrasound scanning. Based on these two interfaces in end-diastole the IVUS measurements are made (Fig. 10.6).

- *Total vessel diameter and area:* Area and diameter confined within external elastic lamina or the media-adventitia interface.
- *Lumen area:* It is the integrated area central to the leading edge echo. The area is confined within the lumen-intima interface.

- Percentage plaque area = $\dfrac{\text{(Total vessel area – lumen area)}}{\text{Total vessel area}} \times 100\%$

Plaque distribution is classified into following categories:

- *Concentric plaque:* Maximum plaque thickness is < 1.3 times of minimal plaque thickness
- *Eccentric plaque:* Maximum plaque thickness is > 1.3 times of minimal plaque thickness. If it is between 1.3 to 1.7, then the eccentricity is moderate. If it is > 1.7, then it is severe.

Plaque Morphology

Studies have compared the ultrasound appearance of plaques with histology in freshly explanted human arteries. The following are the morphological features that are picked up by IVUS *in vivo*:

- *Echo-lucent plaques:* A plaque can be identified by low echogenecity if it is lipid-rich, frequently these lesions exhibit a prominent echogenic border structure at the lumen-intima interface. This may correspond to the anatomic structure of fibrous cap [in unstable lesion the fibrous cap is too thin (< 65 μm) to be resolved by IVUS]. Low echogenecity of plaque may be caused by:
  - Necrosis within the plaque
  - Intramural hemorrhage
  - Thrombus.

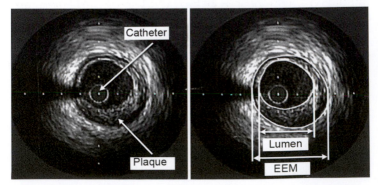

Fig. 10.6: Assessment of plaque by IVUS

Thrombus is usually recognized as an intramural mass, often with a layered, lobulated or pedunculated appearance. But, IVUS cannot really differentiate between acute thrombus and echo-lucent plaque.

- *Echodense plaques:* The plaques have an intermediate echogenicity between echolucent atheromas and echogenic calcified plaques and together with mixed lesions represent the majority of atherosclerotic lesions.
- *Calcified plaques:* Ultrasound imaging has shown significant higher sensitivity and specificity than fluoroscopy in the detection of coronary calcification. Bright echoes within a plaque which demonstrate acoustic shadowing (obstruction of ultrasound penetration) is due to calcium deposit within the plaque. Calcium is classified as deep or superficial, and again depending upon the degree of circumference in which the shadowing is present.
- *Superficial or deep calcium:* The leading edge of the acoustic shadowing appears within the superficial or deep 50% of the atheroma thickness respectively.

The arc of calcium can be measured (in degrees) by using an electronic protractor centered on the lumen.

The length of the calcium deposit can also be measured during pull back.

If, there is superficial calcium more than 270° arc, rotablation would be appropriate for lesion preparation before stenting.

Diagnostic Applications of IVUS

Indeterminate Coronary Artery Lesions

This is particularly important when the lesions are of intermediate (40–70%) severity in presence of mild or atypical symptoms. The gold standard of functional assessment of these lesions is fractional flow reserve, as it accurately defines hemodynamically significant lesions. Many studies have attempted to identify IVUS criteria that are equivalent to fractional flow reserve or noninvasive ischemia testing. Although, IVUS minimum lumen area (MLA) was the parameter best correlated with ischemia, reported thresholds vary with vessel size and it is more correlative in larger (>3.5 mm) arteries than smaller arteries and overall predictive value is moderate, indicating that although it may be acceptable to defer an intervention in selected situations based on MLA size, IVUS should never be used in non-LMCA arteries to justify an intervention. MLA values for ischemia producing lesions (fractional flow reserve < 0.8) are shown in Table 10.3.

Compared to non-LMCA lesions, IVUS determined MLA appears to have better accuracy to predict significant fractional flow reserve in LMCA. IVUS must be performed from both LAD and LCX back to LMCA, (i) to define MLA of LMCA, and (ii) to assess accurately disease in LAD

Table 10.3: IVUS cut-off: non-LMCA arteries

Reference vessel	Minimal lumen area
2.5–3 mm	2.4 mm²
3–3.5 mm	2.7 mm²
>3.5 mm	3.6 mm²

Flow chart 10.1: IVUS cut-off: Non-LMCA arteries

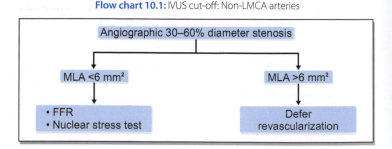

and LCX ostia. An MLA >4 mm² and plaque burden <50% at the LCX ostium is rarely associated with FFR < 0.8 (After single stent crossover). The importance of IVUS is basically to rule out or defer PCI if the cut-off MLA is > 6 mm². If it is less, then it should be supported by other noninvasive tests or clinical history.

It is safe to defer LMCA revascularization with MLA > 6 mm². Additionally, the data confirms that MLA < 6 mm² is clinically significant, correlates with fractional flow reserve < 0.75 and warrant intervention to improve 1 year mortality. In Asian populations, with smaller normal coronary diameters, an MLA cut-off < 4.8 mm² correlates better to reduced FFR < 0.8, while, MLA cut-off < 4.1 mm² with FFR <0.75 (Flow chart 10.1).

There is no data about IVUS criteria of SVG, but it is recommended to use a cut-off point MLA < 4 mm² for graft supplying one artery and MLA < 6 mm² for graft supplying two arteries.

Hazy Lesions

The main finding in the so called hazy lesions is a defect in contrast filling of the coronary arteries. The reasons are:
- Eccentric calcification
- Significant stenosis
- Dissection
- Thrombosis
- Plaque rupture
- Flow phenomenon (inadequate filling of big arteries during dye injection, excepting thrombus)

IVUS can rule out all causes of hazy lesions with reduction in incidence of unnecessary PCI.

Assessing PCI

There are data to suggest that with bare-metal stents, IVUS guided PCI results in a lower target vessel revascularization rate during follow-up. This has been attributed to the improved stent expansion achieved with IVUS guidance compared to angiography alone.

In DES era, the maximal expansion may not be as critical but still important. Recent trials shows, that using IVUS at least in complex PCI can reduce the mortality, (MAIN-COMPARE) early or long-term events (MATRIX) and stent thrombosis (AVIO, PRAVIO and ADAPT-DES) Optimal minimal stent area threshold is smaller in DESs than in BMSs.

It may seem intuitive that strategies to improve poststent areas would decrease adverse events, but there is little data to support this concept in DES era. Furthermore, over aggressive stent sizing and very high pressure postdilatation can result in adverse events, such as vessel perforation, balloon rupture, over-stretch injury and edge dissections. Optimal stent area should be achieved according to reference vessel size.

IVUS measurements of stent length and minimum stent lumen area have influenced the long-term outcome of DES stenting. In a study of 449 patients (543 lesions) who completed 6 months angiographic follow-up after implantation of sirolimus eluting stents, the postprocedural minimum stent lumen area and stent length of IVUS emerged as the only predictors of stent restenosis. IVUS cut-off values that predicted restenosis were a minimum stent lumen of 5.5 mm^2 and a stent length of 40 mm. The use of IVUS in DES era could not come to a conclusion whether TLR is reduced in routine cases of PCI using IVUS, but the reduction of stent thrombosis particularly in complex subsets is apparent in most of the studies when IVUS is being used.

Largest prospective IVUS study so far (ADAPT-DES) done on 3,349 patients undergoing IVUS-guided PCI and 5,234 patients undergoing angiography guided PCI has thrown light into this matter (Tables 10.4 and 10.5).

IVUS guidance improved clinical outcomes both acute (<30 days) and at 1 year and there were:
- 33% reduction in myocardial infarction
- 50% reduction in subacute and late stent thrombosis.

Table 10.4: Relationship between IVUS guidance and clinical outcomes after DES (ADAPT-DES substudy)

1 year outcome	IVUS (n = 3,349)	Angiography (n = 5234)	P value
Definite/probable stent thrombosis	0.6%	1.0%	0.02
Myocardial infarction	2.5%	3.7%	0.002
MACE	3.1%	4.7%	0.006
Greatest benefit present in patients with ACS and complex lesions			

Table 10.5: Stent sizing and area matrix (ADAPT-DES)

Stent diameter	Nominal 100% area (mm^2)	Approx 100% CSA	Nominal 70% area (mm^2)	Approx 70% CSA
2.25	3.95	4	2.78	3
2.5	4.91	5	3.43	3.5
2.75	5.94	6	4.16	4
3.0	7.07	7	4.59	5
3.5	9.62	10	6.73	7
3.75	11.4	11	7.73	8
4.0	12.56	12	8.79	9
4.5	15.90	16	11.13	11

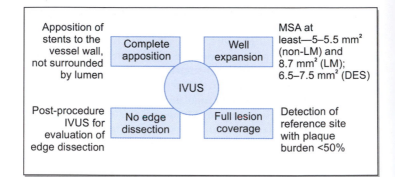

Fig. 10.7: IVUS criteria for optimal stent deployment

- Good apposition of stent struts to the vessel wall such that the stent are not surrounded by lumen
- Only treat major dissections and intramural hematomas, not minor edge dissections.

ADAPT-DES suggests that IVUS guidance may be particularly beneficial among patients with complex lesion characteristics including left main, bifurcations, and multivessel disease, as well as patients with acute coronary syndrome, particularly those patients with STEMI undergoing primary PCI. Whether IVUS, which falls short of differentiating thrombus from other tissue types, is the ideal imaging technology for the assessment of thrombotic lesions remains unclear. In ADAPT-DES, it was found that stent under expansion and/or residual disease at the stent edge, which are known as predictors for early stent thrombosis, may be missed by angiography alone, but ADAPT-DES is not randomized and does not make clear when and how operators decided to use IVUS, leaving the results open to possible selection bias.

The possible IVUS criteria for optimal stent deployment can be summarized in Figure 10.7.

During PCI, IVUS can be used to select stent size, identify optimum proximal and distal stent edge landing zones and select stent length using motorized pullback to measure the distance between proximal and distal landing zones. Optimum landing zones are the largest lumens with the smallest plaque burden in the same coronary artery segment, ideally a plaque burden, less than 50%. These are called reference segments. Using EEM dimension at the reference or at the site of the lesion, will result in over-estimation of the vessel size, since EEM diameter reflect a degree of positive remodeling in most cases. This can result in device oversizing and should be avoided.

So for all practical purposes, few IVUS facts are to be remembered while doing IVUS for optimization of drug-eluting stent deployment.

- Measure proximal and distal reference lumen area
- Measure proximal and distal reference cross-sectional area (CSA)
- Measure the lesion lumen and CSA
- Measure length of the stent
- After deployment, again measure all the relevant areas by IVUS and see whether criteria are met, if not, then use high P. balloon (NC) dilatation.

Criteria for Optimum Drug-eluting Stent Deployment (Fig. 10.8)

- *Stop criteria:* STOP TRIAL (JIC. 2014;26(12):640-46)
  - Distal stent CSA ≥ 60% distal reference CSA
  - Mid stent CSA ≥ 70% distal reference CSA
  - Minimum stent CSA ≥ 70% distal reference CSA
  - Proximal stent CSA ≥ 60% proximal reference chronic stable angina.
- IVUS XPL criteria for stent optimization (JAMA. 2015;314(20))
  - Minimal luminal CSA > lumen cross-sectional area at the distal reference segments.

Guidance for Unprotected LMCA Intervention

IVUS guided strategy in LMCA intervention has shown to reduce 3 years mortality (MAIN-COMPARE). The mechanism of benefit is postulated to be related to reduced rates of sudden cardiac death related to late stent thrombosis. With a single cross-over stenting, a postinternvention ostial LCX MLA ≥ 4 mm² is associated with a restenosis rate of 6% compared with 50% in those with MLA < 4 mm².

The best IVUS MSA criteria that predicted angiographic ISR were 5 mm² for LCX ostium, 6.3 mm² for LAD, 7.2 mm² for polygon of confluence and 8.2 mm² for the proximal LMCA.

Guidance In Chronic Total Occlusion

May be extremely useful in identification of true and false lumen, optimal entry point within chronic total occlusion (CTO cap). Also gives a clue to the true size of the vessel and length of the required stent.

Detection of PCI Complications

1. *Malapposition:* Stent malapposition, synonymous with incomplete stent apposition, is lack of stent-vessel wall contact and is identified

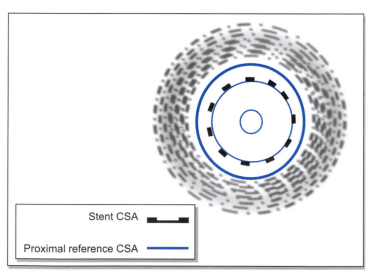

Fig. 10.8: IVUS image

using IVUS as blood speckle behind stent struts not overlying a side branch. Stent malapposition (whether acute or persistent or late and acquired) is common, occurring in 10–20% in IVUS studies, in stable patients and 30–40% in STEMI patients. There is no evidence supporting acute stent malapposition is an important cause of early stent thrombosis.

2. *Edge dissection:* IVUS is more sensitive in detection of dissections as compared to angiography and can accurately determine whether the dissection extends into the wall.

   An IVUS classification of dissection is primarily is based on the depth of the dissection (i.e., intimal, medial or extending to the adventitia). Stent edge dissections are quantitatively and qualitatively evaluated at the proximal and distal reference segments. Effective lumen CSA (lumen CSA – area behind the dissection flap at the site of smallest lumen CSA within the dissection segment), maximum dissection angle and length are measured (Fig. 10.9).

   Residual stent edge dissection, especially those with smaller effective CSA, affects TLR at 1 year follow-up.

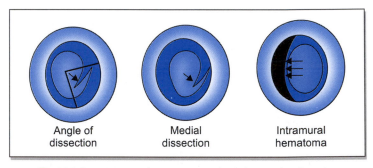

| Angle of dissection | Medial dissection | Intramural hematoma |

Fig. 10.9: Quantitative and quantitative analysis of stent edge dissection

Future perspectives: It is somewhat disconcerting that after more than 20 years of intravascular imaging, there remains a void of convincing data to support its use in routine clinical practice. Intuitively any imaging technique with superior resolution, improve tissue characterization and easier interpretations should advance both diagnosis and treatment. Until then, angiography guided PCI will remain the standard of care which may be supplemented by intracoronary imaging in selected high-risk patients and lesion subsets such as those deriving the greatest benefit in ADAPT-drug eluting stents. But one can always optimize the routine angiography guided PCI procedures with knowledge acquired and learned from studies being performed using IVUS.

Optical Coherence Tomography

Optical coherence tomography (OCT) uses scattering and absorption of near-infrared light. The OCT light source operates on a wave-length range of 1250–1350 nm providing tissue penetration of 1–3 mm and a spatial resolution at the cellular level. It has very high axial and lateral resolution, which provides accurate characterization of plaque morphology and composition in real time, including thin fibrous caps,

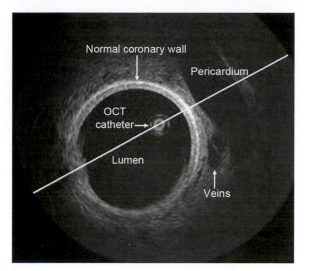

Fig. 10.10: OCT image

lipid pools and fibrocalcific plaques. OCT has better resolution than IVUS, but less power of penetration. OCT is better for looking at fine detail in the near field, around the lumen and stent edges, but is less valuable in imaging plaque size or determining tissue characteristics. The improved spatial resolution compared to IVUS has raised the possibility that OCT could ultimately replace IVUS. However, its limited depth of penetration mitigates its ability to visualize the external elastic lamina, especially in large proximal vessels (Fig. 10.10).

As OCT can delineate the vessel wall more than other intravascular imaging and lower the interobserver variability obtain with intravascular ultrasound. The higher resolution of the method allows for a more automated software segmentation of the lumen with less human input, leading to higher reproducibility.

Diagnostic Intravascular OCT

- *Stable angina:* The size of the blood vessel can be more accurately assessed by OCT, this is particularly helpful in LMCA disease (in shaft and distal bifurcation). Ostial left main is not consistently imaged by intravascular OCT.
- *Acute coronary syndrome:* OCT has 100% sensitivity (versus 33% sensitivity of IVUS) in detection of intravascular thrombus. It is considered as Gold standard for detection of thin cap fibro-atheroma (TCFA).

Lesion Assessment

OCT has high tissue penetration on calcium which allows for assessment of the calcium thickness. Thin, concentric calcium can be fractured by scoring balloons or NC balloons where as thicker calcium should be treated by atherectomy.

Stent Selection

Current metallic stent can be expanded up to an average of 1.5 mm in diameter over their normal size. Stent selection by OCT most often sized to the reference lumen dimensions as the limited penetration of OCT often precludes EEM measurements. Diameter selection with OCT is dictated by the smallest reference vessel diameter, which is usually the distal reference. Depending on the condition of the landing zone, different degrees of diameter oversizing can be applied in "Close to normal" vessels or concentric predominantly fibrotic lesions (oversizing by 0.25–0.5).

When a stent or scaffold is oversized, it should be deployed at nominal pressure. In eccentric calcified or lipid-rich plaque contain distal landing zones, 1:1 size is preferable, in order to avoid edge dissection.

Stent length selection on OCT is determined mostly by volumetric assessment of the lumen area profile and adding a minimum 3 mm to the total length.

Stent Optimization

This is the single most important parameter that has been correlated with clinical outcomes. In order to determine under – expansion, a reference vessel lumen diameter has to be considered. If in any given region of the stented segment, the lumen area is inferior to the reference area, this is considered as underexpansion.

Edge Dissection and Tissue Prolapse

OCT has a very high sensitivity for edge dissection, possibly more than what is clinically relevant. The vast majority of edge dissections heal without clinical consequences. The best situations is to avoid edge dissections by finding a good landing zone and to select an appropriate stent diameter.

The high resolution of OCT detects edge dissection not seen by angiography and even IVUS, although some such disruptions are clinically benign, others may be sinister. The present observation that dissection flap thickness is an important predictor of adverse outcome related to stent thrombosis and restenosis makes pathologic and clinical sense. Bouki and Stefandis (CCI, 2015) showed that edge dissections with a flap thickness > 0.31 mm had significantly decreased event-free survival compared to patients with thinner dissection flap or without any dissection. Interestingly, the longitudinal extension or the flap length was not found to affect prognosis.

In the presence of intramural hematoma should an additional stent be placed to seal the dissection in order to avoid vessel collapse.

Stent Malapposition

Stent malapposition is qualitatively defined as lack of contact of stent struts with the vessel wall in nonbifurcated segments. Significance of malapposition is unknown. A stent that is circumferentially malapposed is always a consequence of stent-vessel size mismatch. In contrast, a focal noncircumferential area of malapposition or even a single malapposed strut is often the result of inability of the stent to conform

Table 10.6: Comparison between IVUS and optical coherence tomography (OCT)

Pathology of vascular wall	IVUS	OCT
Necrotic core	+	++
Thin cap fibroatheroma	–	+++
Thrombus	+	+++
Calcium	+++	++
Stent apposition/expansion	++	+++
Stent dissection	++	+++
Ostial lesion evaluation	++	+

(*Source:* KS Rallaod, S Hampshire. Radcliffe Cardiology, 2015)

on irregularities, typically, due to intravascular calcium and it should not be given much importance (Table 10.6).

Summary of Recommendation [SCAI 2011]

Fractional Flow Reserve

Definitely Beneficial

- In stable angina patients when noninvasive stress imaging is contra-indicated. Fractional flow reserve (FFR) should be used to assess frictional significance of intermediate coronary stenosis (50–70%) and more severe stenosis (<90%). In the later group, about 20% could be hemodynamically insignificant to demand PCI
- In patients with multivessel disease, PCI-guided by FFR measurement improves outcome
- In stable ischemic heart disease patients, medical therapy is indicated for an angiographically intermediate stenosis (LMCA or non-LMCA), when FFR is > 0.80 and PCI required, if FFR < 0.80.

Intravascular Ultrasound

- *Definitely beneficial:* Intravascular ultrasound (IVUS) is an accurate method for determining optimal stent deployment (Complete stent expansion and apposition and lack of edge dissection or other complications after implantation) and the size of the vessel undergoing stent implantation
- *Probably beneficial:* IVUS can be used to appraise the significance of LMCA stenosis and employing a cut-off MLA = 6 mm^2 LIMA cut-off values (Kang et al.)
- *Possibly beneficial:* Can be used to assess plaque morphology.

Optical Coherence Tomography

- *Probably beneficial:* Optimal stent deployment (sizing, apposition and lack of edge dissection) with improved resolution compared with IVUS.
- *Possibly beneficial:* OCT can be useful for assessment of plaque morphology.

Suggested Reading

1. Lotfi A, Jeremias A, Fearson W. Expert consensus statement on the use of FFR, IVUS and OCT. A consensus statement of SCAI. Cath Cardiovascular Intervention. 2014;83:509-18.

2. Witzenbichler B, Machera A, Weisz U. Relationship between IVUS Guidance and Clinical Outcomes after DES (ADAPT-DES Study): Circulation. 2014;29:463-70.

3. FFR and Complex Coronary Pathologic conditions: WK Hau European Heart Journal. 2004;25:723-7.

4. Raber L, Windecker S. IVUS guided PCI: An ongoing Odyssey, Circulation AHA. 2014;129:417-9.

Drugs Used in Cathlab and Mechanical Circulatory Support

■ Siddhartha Bandyopadhyay, Shuvanan Ray

Antiplatelet Agents

They are the cornerstone of the cardiovascular interventions. These agents can be divided into three groups, depending on their mode of action:

- *1st Group:* Cyclooxygenase inhibitor, e.g. Aspirin
- *2nd Group:* ADP receptor antagonists, e.g. Clopidogrel, Prasugrel, Ticagrelor
- *3rd Group:* Glycoprotein IIb/IIa inhibitor.

These agents alone or in combination, prevent pre-, intra- or post-operative cardiovascular adverse events.

Cyclooxygenase Inhibitor

Aspirin: It is the mainstay of treatment in coronary artery disease since the early days of coronary interventions. It irreversibly inhibits Cyclo-oxygenase activity. It is rapidly absorbed at gastrointestinal (GI) tract and peak plasma level is reached within less than 40 minutes of administration. At present, guideline recommendations are as follows:

1. Patients already taking aspirin daily should take 81–325 mg aspirin before PCI.
2. Patients not on aspirin therapy should take non-enteric-coated aspirin 325 mg before PCI.
3. It should be continued indefinitely after PCI.

Adenosine Diphosphate Receptor Antagonists

These agents inhibit platelet activation by binding and inhibiting platelet $P2Y_{12}$ adenosine diphosphate (ADP) receptor. These receptors play critical role in activation and aggregation of platelets. These ADP receptor antagonist can inhibit platelets reversibly (ticagrelor) or irreversibly (clopidogrel, prasugrel, etc.). At present, all three agents are approved for clinical use. Besides these above-mentioned three oral agents, an intravenously given ADP receptor antagonist, cangrelor is also there. But it is still under evaluation and, till now, has not shown any superiority over oral agents.

Clopidogrel

It is a pro-drug and requires activation through two-step reaction involving *CYP450* enzymes. Only 15% of clopidogrel undergoes two-step activation process resulting in slower onset of action and wide variation in bioavailability. Based on the CURRENT-OASIS trial, high-dose clopidogrel regimen of 600 mg loading dose and 150 mg maintenance dose in 1st week, followed by 75 mg maintenance dose can be considered, if prasugrel and ticagrelor are not available or contraindicated.

Prasugrel

It is a third-generation ADP receptor antagonist. Onset of action is rapid, within 1–2 hours and it achieves greater platelet inhibition with fewer drug-drug interactions and less individual variability. It is a pro-drug but activation occurs via more efficient pathway resulting in peak platelet inhibition within 30–60 minutes afterloading dose. It offers more predictable and rapid platelet inhibition than clopidogrel. In diabetic patients with acute coronary syndrome (ACS), prasugrel offers better clinical outcome than clopidogrel. Prasugrel should be considered in patients with stent thrombosis despite proper clopidogrel regimen. It is contraindicated in patients with prior history of TIA or stroke. Loading dose of prasugrel is 60 mg followed by 10 mg daily. Patients >75 years of age and low body weight (<60 kg) should get 60 mg loading dose and reduced maintenance dose of 5 mg daily.

Ticagrelor

Unlike clopidogrel and prasugrel, it inhibits platelets reversibly. Plasma half-life is approximately 6–12 hours. Usual dose is 180 mg loading followed by 90 mg twice daily. PLATO trial showed significant benefit of ticagrelor over clopidogrel in composite ischemic end-point in ACS patients. Ticagrelor is associated with increased rate of adverse effect including dyspnea, increased frequencies of ventricular pause and asymptomatic increase in serum uric acid levels.

Recommendations

1. Aspirin is recommended for all STEMI and Non-ST-segment elevation-acute coronary syndrome (NSTE-ACS) patients without contraindication at an initial oral dose of 150–300 mg and at a maintenance dose of 75–100 mg daily long-term regardless of treatment strategy.
2. A $P2Y_{12}$ inhibitor is recommended in addition to ASA and should be continued over 12 months unless there are contraindications such as excessive bleeding. Options are:
   a. Prasugrel (60 mg loading dose, 10 mg daily dose) in patients when coronary anatomy is known and who are proceeding to PCI.
   b. Ticagrelor (180 mg loading dose, 90 mg twice daily dose) regardless of treatment strategy, including those pretreated with clopidogrel (75 mg once daily), if no contraindication.
   c. In STEMI and NSTE-ACS patients, clopidogrel should only be used if ticagrelor or prasugrel are not available.
   d. In spontaneous coronary artery dissection (SCAD) patients, pretreatment with clopidogrel 600 mg is recommended, once anatomy is known.
   e. Pretreatment with prasugrel in whom coronary artery not known, is not recommended.

Antiplatelet Therapy after Stenting

1. Dual antiplatelet therapy (DAPT) is indicated for at least 1 month after bone-metal stent (BMS) implantation.
2. DAPT therapy is indicated for 6 months after drug-eluting stents implantation in SCAD patients and more than 1 year in ACS patients.
3. GPIIb/IIIa inhibitor should be considered for bailout situation and in thrombotic, no reflow situation.
4. Upstream use of GPIIb/IIIa inhibitor is not recommended in NSTE-ACS patients. In STEMI, upstream use of GPIIb/IIIa inhibitors may be considered in high-risk patients.

Intravenous Glycoprotein IIb/IIIa Inhibitors

Platelet GPIIb/IIIa receptors mediate the final common pathway of platelet aggregation by binding fibrinogen and other adhesive proteins that bridge platelets. Currently, approved three agents are abciximab, eptifibatide and tirofiban. All three inhibitors are given via parenteral route:

Abciximab

Humanized Fab fragment of murine monoclonal antibody against GPIIb/IIIa receptor. Majority of drug is cleared from body within 26 minutes, but because of much slower clearance from the body, its functional half-life is up to 7 days. Dose of abciximab is 250 µg/kg, 10-6 minutes before the procedure followed by IV infusion at 0.125 µg/kg/min for 12 hours. History of any active major bleeding, thrombocytopenia, CVA within 2 years, peptic ulcer disease, uncontrolled hypertension should be taken.

Eptifibatide

It is a peptide molecule. Recommended dose is 180 µg/kg bolus followed by another bolus dose of 180 µg/kg and infusion at the rate of 2 µg/kg/min. Plasma concentration decreases rapidly after stopping infusion. Elimination half-life is 2.5 hours. As majority of the drug is eliminated via renal mechanism a lower infusion rate 1 µg/kg/min is recommended in patients with creatinine clearance less than 50 mL/min. Recovery of platelet aggregation becomes evident within 4 hours of discontinuation of the infusion.

Tirofiban

Another peptide molecule competitively inhibits platelet aggregation mediated by fibrinogen and VW factor. Like eptifibatide, recovery of platelet aggregation occurs within 4 hours of stopping the IV infusion.

Dose: Initial IV bolus 25 µg/kg over 30 minutes, followed by maintenance infusion at the rate of 0.15 µg/kg/min for up to 18 hours. Dose adjustments are needed in case of creatinine clearance less than 50 mL/min. Bolus dose remains same, but infusion rate is lowered at 0.075 µg/kg/min.

Recommendations

- In STEMI, GPIIb/IIIa inhibitors should be considered for bailout on evidence of no reflow or thrombotic complications.
- Upstream of GPIIb/IIIa inhibitors may be used in high-risk patients undergoing transfer for primary PCI
- In NSTE-ACS, GPIIb/IIIa inhibitors should be considered for bailout situation or thrombotic complications.
- In NSTE-ACS, pretreatment with GPIIb/IIIa inhibitors is not recommended in recent guidelines.

Anticoagulant therapy

Anticoagulation is recommended for all patients in addition to antiplatelet therapy during PCI. Most commonly used agents are unfractional heparin (UFH), low-molecular weight heparin (LMWH), Factor Xa inhibitors (Fondaparinux) and direct thrombin inhibitors (Bivalirudin).

Merits and Demerits of Agents

UFH binds to several plasma protein and cell surface protein. This non-specific binding results in variable anticoagulant activity. For which monitoring of therapeutic effect is required. Half-life of UFH is approximately 30 minutes.

Compared to UFH, LMWH binds less avidly with plasma protein and cell surface proteins, resulting in more predictable pharmacokinetics. Laboratory monitoring of LMWH anticoagulant activity is not required, though it can be done by measuring anti-Xa level. After SC injection 90% of the drug is bioavailable and its anti-Xa effect peaks around 3–5 hours of administration. As LMWH is cleared by renal mechanism, drugs accumulate in patients with impaired renal function. In normal renal function, its half-life is around 3–6 hours.

Among direct thrombin inhibitors bivalirudin is most extensively studied. These agents do not require antithrombin. They directly inhibit thrombin-dependent fibrin production and also reduce thrombin-mediated platelet activation and aggregation. Bivalirudin is a synthetic peptide with half-life of 25 minutes. This helps in quick sheath removal. Sheath can be removed 2 hours after stopping the infusion. Though it mostly undergoes hepatic metabolism, it has some dependence on renal excretion. So in patients with severe renal dysfunction, sheath removal should be delayed up to 8 hours.

Previous evidence indicates that bivalirudin provides a moderate benefit over unfractionated heparin (UFH) in patients undergoing primary PCI, but recent studies (HEAT-PPCI) suggest a significant benefit of low-dose heparin over bivalirudin and confirm the acute risk of stent thrombosis associated with bivalirudin. Contrary to the previous trials of heparin versus bivalirudin, stent thrombosis did not catch up in the heparin group during follow-up perhaps because of high rate of potent P2Y12 use. Moreover, no increase in bleeding complications were observed in a predominantly radial approach. Given the high cost of bivalirudin, its future role in PCI is narrowed to patients who are intolerant to UFH.

Recommendations

The anticoagulation is selected accordingly to both ischemic and bleeding risks, according to efficacy–safety profile of the agent (Table 11.1).

In NSTE-ACS, bivalirudin is recommended as alternative to UFH-plus GPIIb/IIIa inhibitors during PCI. For patients who have received UFH, wait for 30 min, then give 0.75 mg/kg IV bolus, then 1.75 mg/kg/hour IV infusion. In patients who have not received prior anticoagulant therapy, dose remains same.

When no GPI is planned, UFH is given at 70–100 mg/kg IV bolus to achieve an ACT of 200–250 sec., if IV GPI is planned, it is given at reduced dose of 50–70 µg/kg to achieve ACT of 200–250 sec.

If patient is on prior treatment of enoxaparin and last dose is administered 8–12 hours earlier, then IV dose 0.3 mg/kg should be given. If there is no history of prior anticoagulant treatment 0.5–0.75 mg/kg should be given. If the last dose was administered within prior 8 hours, no additional enoxaparin should be given.

As present, guidelines are based on OASIS-5 trial, many of the patients of NSTE-ACS will be on fondaparinux. Its bleeding complication are significantly lower than enoxaparin. But due to high incidence of catheter thrombosis in patients treated with fondaparinux alone, full dose of UFH (85 U/kg) must be added during PCI.

Earlier studies on ACS patients receiving conservative treatment demonstrated superiority of enoxaparin over UFH. But more recent studies in the setting of PCI did not find any advantage of enoxaparin over UFH.

Table 11.1: Algorithm suggesting antithrombotic strategies according to bleeding and ischemic risk

Risk	Preloading with	Anticoagulant therapy	Antithrombotic therapy at discharge
Low bleeding risk, low ischemic risk	Aspirin and clopidogrel	Bivalirudin or unfractionated heparin	Aspirin, clopidogrel
Low bleeding risk, high ischemic risk	Aspirin and prasugrel or ticagrelor[a]	Heparin plus a glycoprotein IIb/IIIa inhibitor bivalirudin	Aspirin and prasugrel or ticagrelor; consider low-dose rivaroxaban
High bleeding risk, low ischemic risk	Aspirin and clopidogrel	Bivalirudin	Aspirin and pasugrel or ticagrelor[a]
High bleeding risk, high ischemic risk	Aspirin and clopidogrel, ticagrelor or prasugrel[a]	Bivalirudin	Aspirin, prasugrel or ticagrelor[a]

[a]General considerations to choose between prasugrel or ticagrelor.

Consider:
Low-dose prasugrel (5 mg) and hybrid regimens with prasugrel or ticagrelor for 30 days before switching to clopidogrel

STEMI: Prasugrel
Non-ST elevation ACSs: Ticagrelor
Prior stroke, < 60 kg, > 75 years, creatinine clearance <60 mL/min: Ticagrelor instead of prasugrel

No-reflow Phenomenon

It describes the persistence of reduced flow and associated failed myocardial reperfusion despite removal of mechanical coronary occlusion. It is mainly seen in acute myocardial infarction following PCI or thrombolytic revascularization. It is also seen in PCI on saphenous venous grafts or native coronary vessels in the setting of unstable angina.

Mechanisms and mediators of no-reflow phenomenon remains speculative. Potential mechanisms are vasospasm, distal embolization of thrombus or other debris, oxygen-free radical-mediated endothelial injury and capillary plugging.

Management (Flow chart 11.1)

The optimal treatment of no-reflow phenomenon is unknown. As it occurs in a variety of clinical settings, so it is likely to have more than one mechanism. It is important to remember that no-reflow phenomenon is a diagnosis of exclusion. High-grade residual stenosis due to flow limiting dissection, thrombus, and stenosis should be systematically excluded since their treatment and outcome are generally more favorable than those of no-reflow.

1. *Reverse superimposed spasm:* Intracoronary nitroglycerin (200–800 µg) rarely has any effect on no-reflow, but may reverse superimposed spasm and should be used in all cases.
2. Exclude coronary dissection.
3. *Administer intracoronary calcium antagonist:* It is the most important strategy of no-reflow. Intracoronary administration of verapamil (100–200 µg, total dose up to 1.0–1.5 mg) or diltiazem (0.5–2.5 mg bolus, total dose up to 5–10 mg) has been shown to reverse no-reflow in 65–95% cases. Resolution of no-reflow 3–4 times is more likely, if verapamil was administered.

    In one report, resolution of no-reflow was 3–4 times more likely if drugs are administered in distal vascular bed. Although high-grade AV block is unusual following intracoronary calcium antagonist, but temporary pacemaker should be readily available. Hypotension caused by no-reflow is not a contraindication to intracoronary calcium channel blockers. Adjunctive therapy with intra-aortic balloon pump (IABP), pressors should be started.
4. *Consider GPIIb/IIIa antagonist:* Use of potent platelet receptor antagonist for preventing or reversing no-reflow is controversial. Some studies suggest benefit, other studies in vein graft do not.
5. Treat distal embolization.
6. Intracoronary adenosine, sodium nitroprusside:
    Potent coronary vasodilators have been used to treat some refractory no-reflow. Intracoronary adenosine 10–20 µg is attractive, because it inhibits WBC function and inhibits free radical formation and endothelial injury.

    Intracoronary nitroprusside 10–50 µg is particularly helpful in the setting of acute myocardial infarction or in vein graft intervention.

Flow chart 11.1: Management of no-reflow phenomenon

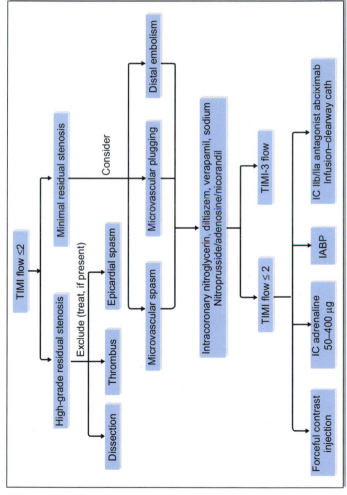

Vasoactive Drugs in Cathlab (Table 11.2)

They can be divided into two broad groups:
1. Vasodilators
2. Vasoconstrictors

Vasodilators

Types: Endothelium-dependent vasodilators—act via healthy endothelium

Endothelium-independent vasodilators—act directly on the vascular smooth muscle cells (VSMCs)

No donors: NTG, nitroprusside

Calcium-channel blockers

Adenosine

Indications:
- Vascular spasm (coronary or non-coronary vessels)
- Slow flow/no reflow phenomenon
- Induction of hyperemia (FFR)

Nitroglycerin (NTG):
- Acts directly on the vascular smooth muscle cells.
- Dilates both coronary and non-coronary vessels.
- Venodilator (decreases preload)
- Commonly used in cathlab to treat hypertension, prevent and treat arterial spasm
- Dosage: 100–400 µg
- It can cause exaggerated hypotension in volume depletion state, RV infarction and volume-dependent pathology like restrictive cardiomyopathy
- Concomitant use with sildenafil is contraindicated.

Sodium nitroprusside:
- Coronary and peripheral arterial vasodilator
- Venodilator
- Mainly used in slow flow/no reflow
- Hypertensive crisis
- Dosage: Intracoronary: 25–200 µg
  Intravenous infusion: 3–200 µg/kg/min

Calcium-channel blockers:

Verapamil: Used in cathlab for:
- Coronary no reflow
- To prevent radial artery spasm

Dose: 50–200 µg intracoronary

Complications: AV nodal block
  Myocardial depression

Diltiazem: Less approved indication as vasodilator in cathlab
- Commonly used in no-reflow
- Dose: 50–100 µg intracoronary; upto 5 mg
- Complications: AV block, sinus arrest
- Less of negative ionotrope compared to verapamil

Adenosine:
- Causes maximum coronary vasodilatation with only mild fall in BP, self-limiting bradycardia for 5–10 seconds.
- Treatment for no-reflow phenomenon
- Induction of hyperemia in FFR
- Dosage: Left coronary—30–90 µg/right coronary—10–50 µg

Table 11.2: Ionotropic and vasopressor drug names, clinical indications for therapeutic use, standard dose range, receptor binding (catecholamines), and major clinical side effects

Drug	Clinical indication	Dose range	Receptor binding				Major side effects
			a1	b1	b2	DA	
Catecholamines							
Dopamine	• Shock (cardiogenic, vasodilatory) • Heart failure • Symptomatic bradycardia unresponsive to atropine or pacing	2.0 to 20 µg kg^{-1} min^{-1} (max 50 µg kg^{-1} min^{-1})	+++	++++	++	+++++	• Severe hypertension (especially in patients taking nonselective β-blockers) • Ventricular arrhythmias • Cardiac ischemia • Tissue ischemia/gangrene (high doses or due to tissue extravasation)
Dobutamine	• Low CO (decompensated HF, cardiogenic shock, sepsis-induced myocardial dysfunction) symptomatic bradycardia unresponsive to atropine or pacing	2.0 to 20 µg kg^{-1} min^{-1} (max 40 µg kg^{-1} min^{-1})	+	+++++	+++	N/A	• Tachycardia • Increased ventricular response rate in patients with atrial fibrillation • Ventricular arrhythmias, cardiac ischemia • Hypertension (especially nonselective β-blocker patients) hypotension
Norepinephrine	• Shock (vasodilatory, cardiogenic)	0.01 to 3 µg kg^{-1} min^{-1}	+++++	+++	++	N/A	• Arrhythmias • Bradycardia • Peripheral (digital) ischemia • Hypertension (especially) nonselective β-blocker patients)

Contd...

Contd...

Drug	Clinical indication	Dose range	Receptor binding				Major side effects
			a1	b1	b2	DA	
Epinephrine	• Shock (cardiogenic, vasodilatory) cardiac arrest • Bronchospasm/anaphylaxis • Symptomatic bradycardia or heart block unresponsive to atropine or pacing	*Infusion:* 0.01 to 0.10 µg kg⁻¹ min⁻¹ *Bolus:* 1 mg IV every 3 to 5 min (max 0.2 mg/kg) IM: (1:1000): 0.1 to 0.5 mg (max 1 mg)	+++++	++++	+++	N/A	• Ventricular arrhythmias • Severe hypertension resulting in cerebrovascular hemorrhage • Cardiac ischemia • Sudden cardiac death
Isoproterenol	• Bradyarrhythmias (especially torsade de pointes) • Brugada syndrome	2 to 10 µg/min	0	+++++	+++++	N/A	• Ventricular arrhythmias • Cardiac ischemia • Hypertension • Hypotension
Phenylephrine	• Hypotension (vagally mediated, medication-induced) • Increases MAP with AS and hypotension • Decreases LVOT gradient in HCM	*Bolus:* 0.1 to 0.5 mg IV every 10 to 15 min *Infusion:* 0.4 to 9.1 µg kg⁻¹ min⁻¹	+++++	0	0	N/A	• Reflex bradycardia • Hypertension (especially with nonselective β-blockers) • Severe peripheral and visceral vasoconstriction • Tissue necrosis with extravasation
Vasopressin	• Shock (vasodilatory, cardiogenic) • Cardiac arrest	*Infusion:* 0.01 to 0.1 U/min (common fixed dose 0.04 U/min) *Bolus:* 40 U IV bolus	V1 receptors (vascular smooth muscle) V2 receptors (renal collecting, duct system)				• Arrhythmias • Hypertension • Decreased CO (at doses > 0.4 U/min) • Cardiac ischemia • Severe peripheral vasoconstriction causing ischemia (especially skin) • Splanchnic vasoconstriction

Vasoconstrictors

Catecholamines

Epinephrine:
- Balanced alpha (α) and beta (β) agonist
- *Indications:* Shock, cardiac arrest (asystole, PEA, VF), anaphylaxis
- *Dosage:* Shock—2–10 µg/min IV; CPR—1 mg every 3 minutes
- Causes tachycardia, increased oxygen demand, increased SVR, BP, arrhythmia.

Norepinephrine:
- Alpha (α) and beta (β) agonist
- *Indications:* Shock refractory to other sympathomimetics, low SVR states
- *Dosage:* Shock—0.5–30 µg/min IV
- Causes ischemia, arrhythmia.

Phenylephrines:
- Pure alpha (α) agonist with minimal beta (β) effect. More long-acting than epinephrine
- *Indications:* Hypotension
- Given as bolus or IV infusion, it causes marked increase in BP with minimal chronotropic effect. May cause reflex bradycardia that can be blocked with atropine.
- *Dosage:* Shock—100 µg bolus (for hypotension).

Isoproterenol:
- Pure beta (β_2) agonist—Not a pressor
- *Indications:* Resistant bradycardia that has failed to respond to atropine and dopamine
- *Dosage:* 2–10 µg/min IV
- Causes marked tachycardia, ionotropic state of heart, decreases DBP and SVR
- Very difficult to titrate dose.

Dopamine:
- *Dose-dependent effects:*
  - 2–5 µg/kg/min—renal and peripheral vasodilator
  - 5–10 µg/kg/min—β_1 agonist—increases contractility
  - 10–20 µg/kg/min—alpha (α)—adrenergic effect.
  - *Indications:* Hypotension, poor tissue perfusion, bradycardia

Vasopressin:
- Causes less direct coronary and cerebral vasoconstriction than catecholamine.
- Dose dependent increase in systemic vascular resistance (SVR) and reflexive increase in vagal tone.
- Directly influences attenuation of NO production and reverses adrenergic receptor downregulation.
- Pressor effects relatively preserved during hypoxic and acidotic conditions.
- *Dosage:*
  - *Infusion:* 0.01 to 0.1 units/min (common fixed dose 0.04 units/min)
  - *Bolus:* 40 unit IV.

Hypotension during PCI (Flow chart 11.2)

Life-threatening hypotension during PCI results from acute bleeding, coronary perforation with cardiac tamponade, arrhythmia, contrast or medication-induced anaphylaxis, no reflow phenomenon, coronary spasm and new thrombus formation. These could occur unexpectedly and may cause fatal outcome.

Vasopressors are generally indicated for a:
- Decrease of SBP ≥30 mm Hg from baseline
- Arterial systolic pressure <80 mm Hg
- Mean arterial pressure <60 mm Hg
- When either condition results in end-organ dysfunction due to hypoperfusion.

Hypovolemia should be corrected prior to institution of vasopressor therapy. These drugs should be used in lowest effective dose and actually they act as the 'pharmacologic bridge' to definitive intervention.

Mechanical Circulatory Support

Heart is the organ which maintains circulation and perfusion of the body through its hemodynamic effects. In acute decompensated heart failure, circulatory failure sets in, blood pressure drops and congestion takes place in distal vascular beds. During complex PCI, maintenance of hemodynamics is the key to success. The goal is often to take over the work, partly or wholly, of a struggling heart, minimize ongoing ischemic damage (especially in acute myocardial infarction) and promote stable hemodynamic state of systemic pressure and perfusion without the need for deleterious vasopressors and inotropes. By resting the heart and simultaneously ensuring end-organ perfusion, the patient returns to an autonomous cardiovascular state with minimum decline in cardiac or end-organ function and potentially improve survival.

Flow chart 11.2: Hypotension during PCI

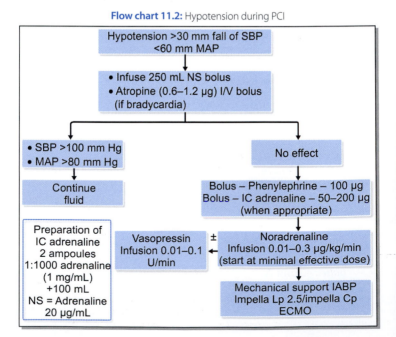

Fundamentals of Ventricular Mechanics

Events occurring during single cardiac cycle are depicted by ventricular pressure-volume loops (PVLs) (Fig. 11.1).

The loop is bounded by the end-systolic pressure volume relationship (ESPVR), which is reasonably linear with slope E_{es} (end-systolic elastance) and volume axis intercept V_o, and end-diastolic pressure-volume relationship (EDPVR) which is nonlinear (Fig. 11.2).

Actual position and shape of the loop depends on the ventricular preload and the afterload. At the organ level, preload can be defined as either end-diastolic pressure (EDP) or the end-diastolic volume (EDV). Afterload is determined by the hemodynamic properties of the vascular system against which the ventricle contracts, and it is more simply indexed by the total peripheral resistance and is depicted in the pressure–volume plane by the effective arterial elastance (E_a) line which cuts the volume axis at the EDV point and intersects the ESPVR at the ventricular end-systolic pressure volume point of loop. EDPVR is nonlinear and is difficult to assess in practice. We take a simpler index called ventricular Capacitance, the volume at a specified filling pressure. This differentiates between systolic and diastolic heart failure. The index used is V30, the volume at an LV filling pressure is elevated (Fig. 11.3).

Research work shows that LV pressure-volume area (PVA) provides the strongest index of oxygen consumption per beat. PVA is the area on the pressure volume diagram bounded by the end-systolic and end-diastolic pressure volume relationship and the systolic portion of the pressure volume curve. In brief, PVA is equal to the external stroke-work (SW) plus the residual energy stored with the myocardium at the end of a beat, also referred to as potential energy (PE). Thus, PVA = SW + PE (Fig. 11.4).

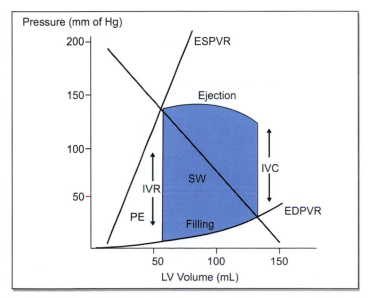

Fig. 11.1: ESPVR and EDPVR shifts with changes in ventricular contractility and diastolic properties. PVA = Pressure volume area is the total mechanical work by ventricle, which correlates closely with total myocardial oxygen consumption per beat

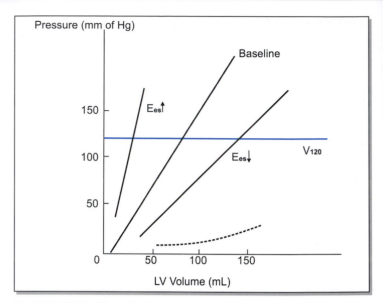

Fig. 11.2: ESPVR shifts with changes in ventricular contractility which can be a combination of changes in E_{es} and V_o. Change in contractility is indexed by V_{120}, the Volume at which ESPVR intersects 120 mm Hg

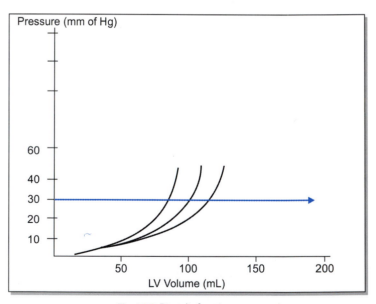

Fig. 11.3: Diastolic function curve

Heart extracts more oxygen from blood than any other organ in the body, attaining arterial-venous oxygen content differences of more than 10–12 mL O_2/100 mL of blood, with typical oxygen content of 20 mL O_2/100 mL of blood. Therefore, under conditions of increased myocardial demand, heart responds majorly by increasing the coronary blood flow.

The rate of coronary blood flow is governed by the principles of fluid dynamics, such that the flow is directly related to the pressure difference

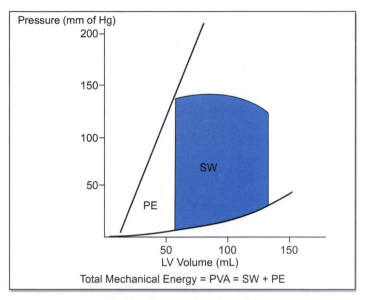

Fig. 11.4: Pressure volume loop of LV

across the vascular bed and inversely related to coronary vascular resistance. As coronary blood flow mainly occurs during diastole, the flow is increased when mean arterial pressure (MAP) is increased and when end diastolic pressure of left ventricle decreases.

So, to summarize, the basic concept is to ensure a stable physiological acceptable.

- Mean arterial pressure (MAP)
- Cardiac output (CO)
- End-diastolic pressure of left ventricle (LVEDP)
- Myocardial oxygen consumption (MVO$_2$)

Recently, a parameter called cardiac power output (CPO) has been explored. It is defined as cardiac output multiplied by mean arterial pressure (Divided by 451 to convert units to watts). It has shown individual association and predictive power in many acute myocardial dysfunctional states.

CPO<0.6 maximized sensitivity and specificity in predicting worsening heart failure, while a CPO cut-point of <0.53 proved predictive of mortality in cardiogenic shock.

Circulatory support strategies help in choosing amongst available mechanical devices which are described in Table 11.3.

Who Requires Mechanical Circulatory Support?

For high-risk PCI requiring MCS, one should consider 3 factors carefully:

1. *Patient-related factors:* Patients presenting with severe heart failure who have been recently stabilized may develop overt heart failure during PCI. Such patients, therefore, benefit from stabilizing effect of an MCS.
2. *Clinical factors:* This includes clinically unstable patients, like those who present with acute myocardial infarction with large infarct areas, cardiogenic shock, acute coronary syndrome with poorly tolerated

Table 11.3: Strategies of circulatory support
(Burkoff & Naidu, CCI. 2012;80:816-29)

Strategy	Therapy/Device	Mechanism	Comments
Medical management	Inotropes	↑ Contractility ↑ Heart rate	
Counterpulsation	IABP	Pressure augmentation	↑ Diastolic pressure ↓ Systolic aortic pressure, ↓ PCWP, No active flow
Extracorporeal bypass heart pump	Tandem heart	LA → AO flow	Indirectly unloads LV by decompressing LA. Up to 4 L/min flow (Retrograde)
	ECMO	RA → AO flow	Provides oxygenation. No LV unloading. Up to 5 L/min flow (Retrograde)
Intracorporeal transvalvular Heart pump	Impella – 2.5–5	LV → AO flow	Directly unloads LV. 2.5 L/min flow (Antegrade), 5 L/min flow (Antegrade)

malignant arrhythmias or acute decompensated heart failure. These people basically require stabilization by an MCS before PCI.

3. *Lesion-specific variables:* Patients with any lesion supplying large area of myocardium and/or a lesion in a last remaining conduit are at high risk during PCI, because any complication may lead to catastrophic consequences from LV dysfunction to cardiogenic shock (Tables 11.6 and 11.7).

Taken together, patients are considered high risk when a combination of all 3 variables produce a picture of a patient who might benefit from MCS during PCI. In most cases, baseline LV dysfunction or clinical instability is a linchpin of the concept of high risk, with anatomic lesion-specific variables which are also considered during final decision for or against MCS (Tables 11.3 and 11.4).

Therapy Comparisons

Support therapy can be classified as: (1) Pharmacological, and (2) Mechanical.

The mechanical support may be basically of four types:

1. Counter-pulsation
2. Percutaneous RA to arterial support (ECMO)
3. Percutaneous LA to arterial pumps
4. Percutaneous LV to aorta pumps

Pharmacological Support Therapy

Most commonly used and is the first-line therapy which consists of the use of inotropic medications and/or vasopressors to return the systemic hemodynamics quickly to more reasonable levels. (Fig. 11.5)

Table 11.4: Contraindications and complications of MCS (Atkinson. JACC, 2016;9(9))

	IABP	Impella	Tandem heart	VA-ECMO
Contraindications	• Moderate-to-severe AR • Severe peripheral vascular disease • Aortic disease	• LV thrombus • Mechanical aortic valve (AVA <0.6) • Moderate-to-severe AR • Severe peripheral vascular disease • Contraindications to anticoagulation	• Severe peripheral vascular disease • HIT • DIC • Contraindications to anticoagulation • LA thrombus • VSD • Moderate-to-severe AR	• Contraindications to anticoagulation • Moderate-to-severe AR • Severe peripheral vascular disease
Complications	• Stroke • Limb ischemia • Vascular trauma • Balloon rupture • Thrombocytopenia • Acute kidney injury • Bowel ischemia • Infection	• Device migration • Device thrombus • Limb ischemia • Vascular trauma • Infection • Stroke	• Air embolism • Thrombombolism • Device dislodgement • Cardiac tamponade • Limb ischemia • Vascular trauma • Infection • Stroke	• Bleeding • Vascular trauma • Limb ischemia • Compartment syndrome • Acute kidney injury • Thromboembolism • Air embolism • Infection • Stroke
Bleeding/Hemolysis	+	++	++	++
Vascular complications	+	++	+++	++++

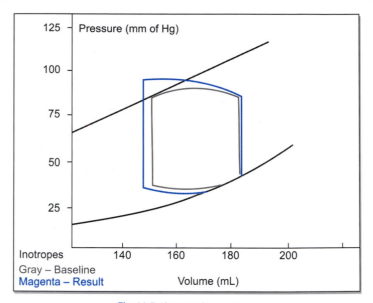

Fig. 11.5: Pharmacologic support

Mechanical Support Therapy

- *Counterpulsation (IABP):* Does not directly pump blood but relies on the native heart to provide forward flow. It is typically used in addition to inotropic drug therapy. Diastolic augmentation improves coronary blood flow, but does not result in substantial improvement in cardiac output. Systemic flow augmentation is still accomplished at the expense of increasing native cardiac work and oxygen consumption. Despite afterload reduction, this increases myocardial oxygen consumption and demand (Fig. 11.6).
- *Percutaneous RA to arterial support (ECMO):* RA–Arterial bypass pump or extracorporeal life support (ECMO) provides better systemic hemodynamic support but crippled by the disadvantage of moving further away from the ventricle which needs to be unloaded.

   So, it leads to larger PVA (pressure-volume area) and MVO$_2$ (myocardial oxygen consumption), both due to increased preload and afterload. More cardiac output and CPO is gained in expense of increased LVEDP (Fig. 11.7).
- *LA-Arterial Bypass Pump:* Tandem heart–LA to Aorta Strategy reduced EDP and significantly increased CO (Cardiac Output), CPO (Cardiac Power Output) and MAP (Mean Arterial Pressure), but PVA remains same or is slightly increased over the baseline. MVO$_2$ (Myocardial Oxygen Consumption) increased despite increased oxygen delivery (Fig. 11.8).
- *LV to Aorta Pumps:* IMPELLA–Continuous pumping of blood directly from LV, independent of phase of cardiac cycle, results in loss of the normal iso-volumic periods of the cycle. This transforms the pressure-volume loops from its normal trapezoid form to a triangular form. Unlike other forms of supports, removal of blood from the LV is not dependent on the ejection through the aortic valve. As pump flow rate increases, the LV becomes increasingly unloaded (progressive leftward shift of P-V Loops). PE (potential

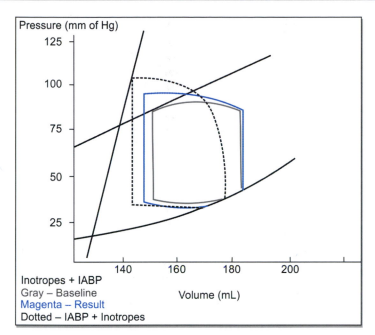

Fig. 11.6: Overall effect: Raised MAP (Mean arterial pressure), Raised HR (Heart rate), Raised CPO (Cardiac power output) and CO (Cardiac output), Raised (Myocardial oxygen consumption) MVO_2

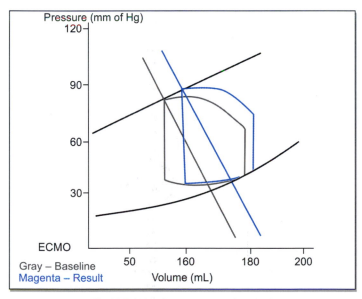

Fig. 11.7: Hemodynamic support by ECMO

energy) decreases, and there is marked decrease in PVA (Pressure-Volume Area) and MVO_2 (Myocardial Oxygen Consumption). At the same time, arterial pressure increases, such that the peak LV pressure and arterial pressure are increasingly dissociated. This will reduce LA pressure and wedge pressure (Figs 11.9A and B).

The hemodynamic effects of all these pumps are summarized in Table 11.5.

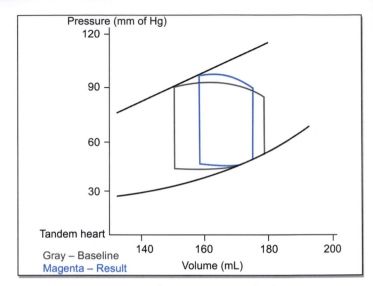

Fig. 11.8: Hemodynamic support—tandem heart

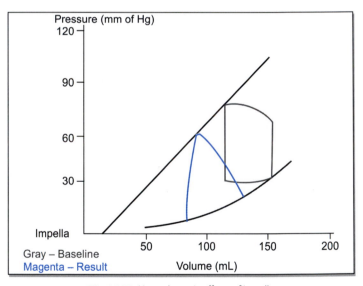

Fig. 11.9A: Hemodynamic effects of Impella

How to Select a Device?

In an emergent patient, shortening the time required to unload the LV and stabilize systemic hemodynamics while reducing PCWP is of paramount importance. The earlier the device can modulate hemodynamics, lesser myocardium will be at risk and smaller will be the risk of end-organ failure, as well as the risk of emergent intubation or life-threatening arrhythmias. So a device which can be easily and rapidly placed in cathlab which provides all these hemodynamic effects rapidly and which does not require excessive maintenance and surgical or specialized teams to look after will be a device of choice (Flow charts 11.3 and 11.4).

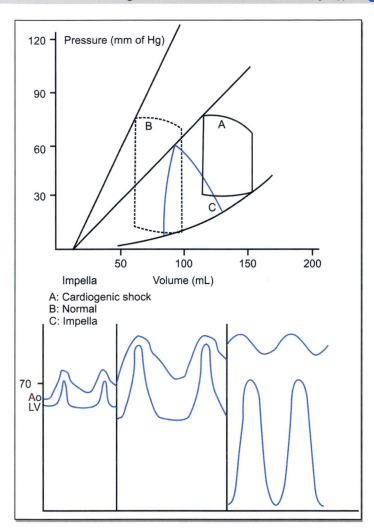

Fig. 11.9B: Hemodynamic support by Impella

Table 11.5: Hemodynamic effects of circulatory supports

	Afterload	Heart rate	PCWP	AOP	CO	CPO	MVO₂
Inotropes	↑↑	↑	—	↑	↑	↑	↑
IABP + Inotropes	↓	↑	↓	↑	↑↑	↑↑	↑
Tandem Heart	↑↑	—	↓↓	↑↑	↑↑	↑↑↑	—
Impella 2.5	↓	—	↓↓	—	↑↑	↑↑↑	↓↓
VA-ECMO	↑↑↑	—	—	↑↑	↑↑	↑↑	—

Abbreviations: PCWP, pulmonary capillary wedge pressure; AOP, aortic pressure; CO, cardiac output; CPO, cardiac power output; MVO₂, myocardial oxygen consumption; ECMO, extracorporeal membrane oxygenation

Table 11.6: High-risk PCI

Clinical	• LVEF <35% • Electrical Instability • CCF
Comorbidities	• Severe AS • Severe MR • Chronic obstructive pulmonary disease • Chronic kidney disease • Diabetes mellitus • Peripheral vascular disease • Age >75 years • Acute coronary syndrome
Coronary anatomy	• Last patent artery • UPLMN (unprotected left main coronary artery) • 3-vessel disease with SYNTAX >33 • Vessel supplying >40% of myocardium • Distal left main bifurcation disease

Flow chart 11.3: High-risk patients (SCAI, 2015)

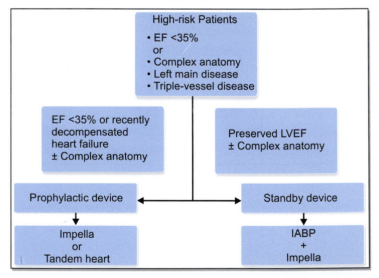

Table 11.7: Cardiogenic shock spectrum

Stage of shock	Clinical	Hemodynamics
Pre/Early shock	• SBP <100 mm of Hg • HR: 70–100 /min • Normal lactate • Normal mental state • Cool extremities	• CI – 2–2.2 • PCWP <20 mm of Hg • LVEDP < 20 mm of Hg • CPO >1 W Vasopressors 0–1, low dose
Shock	• SBP <90 mm of Hg • HR >100 /min • Lactate: 2–4 • Altered mental state • Cool extremities	• CI – 1.5–2 • PCWP >20 mm of Hg • LVEDP > 20 mm of Hg • CPO <1 W Vasopressors 1, moderate dose
Severe Shock	• SBP <90 mm of Hg • HR >120/min • Lactate >4 • Obtunded mental state • Cool extremities	• CI – <1.5 • PCWP >30 mm of Hg • LVEDP >30 mm of Hg • CPO <0.6 W Vasopressors 2+, high dose

Flow chart 11.4: MCS after Cardiac Arrest (JACC, 2016)

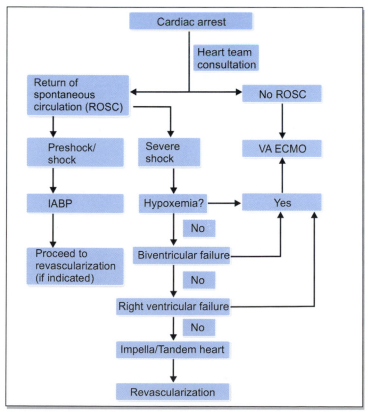

Suggested Reading

1. Dangas GD, Sharma SK, IF Palacios. Interventional Pharmacology. Clinics Review Articles. 2013;2(4).
2. Heechoi j, Kook – Jin Chun. Usefulness of Intracoronary epinephrine in severe hypotension during PCI: Korean Circulation Journal. 2013;43:739.
3. Prognosis and treatment of cardiogenic shock complicating acute myocardial Infarction. *www.uptodate.com*, Aug 12, 2014.
4. Unfractionated heparin outperforms bivalirudin in PPCI. *www.jwatch.org* (NEJM), August 2014.

Difficult Subsets
Remember KISS (Keep it Simple Stupid)!

■ Shuvanan Ray

Bifurcation Stenosis Percutaneous Coronary Intervention

Coronary bifurcation are prone to develop atherosclerotic plaque because of turbulent blood flow and high shear stress, and these lesions account for 15–20% of the total number of percutaneous coronary intervention (PCI) performed. A true coronary bifurcation lesion consists of more than 50% diameter obstruction of the main vessel and the side branch (SB) (Fig. 12.1).

In the balloon angioplasty era, the bifurcation lesions were a relative contraindication; but with advent of stents and new techniques (Provisional stenting) and later drug-eluting stents and selective 2-stent techniques (Crush, Culotte, T&V), bifurcation lesions are being successfully treated with excellent long-term results.

Anatomy and Classification

Recent pathological data confirm that in bifurcation stenosis the main atherosclerotic burden affects sides as well as upper and lower vessels—the carina remains unaffected.

PCI of bifurcation stenosis depends on involvement of side branch, size of side branch and angle between the main vessel and SB, the carina almost never gets involved.

Depending upon SB involvement, many classifications of bifurcation stenosis evolved. Of them, the most recent and most simple is Medina classification (Figs 12.2 and 12.3). There is only one objection to this scheme which is, that it does not account for angulations, which significantly contributes in procedural success.

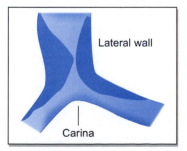

Fig. 12.1: Atherosclerosis affects bifurcation points but spares carina

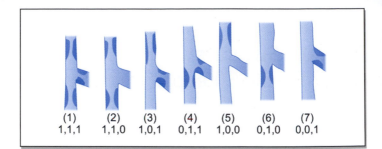

Fig. 12.2: Medina classification system

D	C	F	G	A	B	E	Duke (Modified)
I-A	I-B	II-A	III-A	II-B	III-B	IV	Safian
1	2	-	4	3	4a	4b	Lefevre
I	-	-	III	IV	II	IV	Sanborn
L	S	2	Im	Is	V	T	Movahed
3	2A	2B	2C	1A	1B	1C	Staico-Feres

Fig. 12.3: Bifurcation stenosis—Classification

In bifurcation anatomy Finet et al. proposed a law, which has been validated by several other studies. According to this law, the ratio between the mother vessel diameter and the sum of the daughter vessel diameter (DM/D_1+D_2) is constant and is about 0.68 ± 0.066. If two diameters are known it is possible to derive the diameter of the third vessel using the formula.

Strategies: Nine meta-analyses dedicated to the outcome of coronary bifurcation lesions have been published. They reported similar results with occurrence of midterm clinical events associated with provisional SB stenting VS dual-stenting strategies, namely, no difference in mortality, TLR or definite stent thrombosis rates. The two main randomized studies (Nordic & BBC one) were included in a meta-analysis of individual data. This meta-analysis confirmed the benefit of simple strategy compared to elective double stenting in all prespecified subgroups. In addition, single stent strategy was associated with a significant reduction in procedural time, X-ray exposure and contrast media volume. Despite the clinical trial reports one stent strategy for bifurcation has several limitations (access to the SB, rewiring and crossing trans-strut to SB with stent) and, therefore, elective 2-stent strategy is useful in certain situations of bifurcation stenosis. If the SB is large enough (> 2.75 mm) with a sufficient territory distribution to justify stent implantation and if the SB has long disease starting from the ostium or if the SB comes out at an odd angle from MB which is difficult to access, elective 2-stent strategy should be the choice.

Techniques (Flow chart 12.1)

Guide catheter selection: Usually large bore 7 F or 8 F extra back-up Guide catheters are selected. For bifurcation stenting, usually good

Flow chart 12.1: Bifurcation (1:1:1) stenting

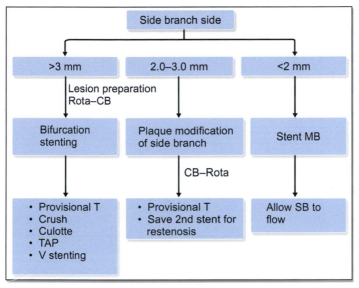

back-up support is required which will be provided by the extra back-up guide catheters. Judkins can be used in special cases, but they should be maneuvered actively to increase support. Large bore catheters are required which will enable two balloons, stents as well as Flextome or Rota burrs to cross easily. Chance of intertwining of wires is less with large bore catheters.

Guidewire technique: Two guidewires to be placed in two branches. Rule is to put the wire in difficult artery first, otherwise there will be entanglement of the wire causing balloon or stent delivery difficult. If there is entanglement of the wires, remove the wire from the straighter vessel and again reintroduce without torquing as much as possible.

Plaque modification: Ostial lesions and bifurcation lesions sometimes become highly fibrotic and calcified. Opening the lesions nicely is the key for good stent expansion and successful stenting procedure. Cutting balloon, scoring balloon or angiosculpt balloons are recommended for moderately calcified and fibrotic lesions. Cutting balloons (Flextome) are better for calcific lesions but they are slightly bulkier than other scoring balloons. In calcified lesions (Calcification arc > 270°) rotational atherectomy is essential for lesion dilatation and hence stent delivery and expansion. In other words, complete opening of the arteries before stenting is essential for a good bifurcation stenting. Risk of stent under expansion should be avoided completely.

Stenting Procedures

1. **Provisional stenting (Fig. 12.4):**
   Candidates are:
   1. SB > 2 mm and easily accessible
   2. Either free of disease or minimally or only ostial disease
   3. Not requiring predilatation of SB or if predilated should not have visible dissection
   4. SB-MB angle < 90°.

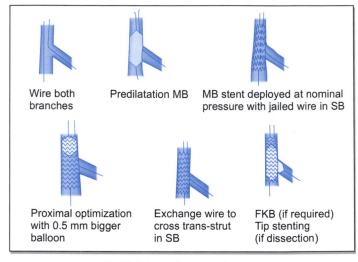

Fig. 12.4: Steps of provisional stenting

Facts to be remembered before doing provisional stenting:

- A stepwise provisional side branch stenting strategy with drug-eluting stents in suitable bifurcation lesions is preferable to elective double stenting in almost 70–80% of cases.
- Jailed wire strategy should be used in all cases.
- Predilatation of the side branch ideally should be avoided before putting stent in main branch. Predilatation may cause:
  1. Dissection of SB ostium or
  2. Promoting proximal trans-strut crossing after MB stent deployment.
- Main branch stent design should allow access and offer optimal plaque scaffolding. A drug-eluting stent with an open cell design or with good stent cell circumference should be selected.
- SB rewiring after MB stenting should be done through the distal strut closest to the flow divider. If a proximal strut is crossed, dilatation (dilatation even with FKB) can distort MB stent, so this should be avoided. If there is a suspicion that a proximal strut is crossed, rewiring of a distal strut should be tried. Proximal optimization of the MB stent a few mm above the flow divider with a 0.5 mm bigger balloon will help the wire to cross distal strut easily.
- Provisional stenting should not be done in severely angulated SB and/or severe ostial involvement or long lesion in SB.

Elective Double Stenting (Flow chart 12.2)

Many techniques using 2-stent to treat bifurcation lesions evolved but no one technique so far, could satisfy every situation. Techniques and strategies should be worked out before the procedure by observing the angiogram very carefully. The type of bifurcation lesions, size of the arteries proximal and distal to the lesion, the length of the proximal artery (in case of LMCA bifurcation), the angle between the bifurcating branches all are necessary for making a strategy. Integrating all the factors, a simplified scheme can be worked out which suits most of the bifurcation lesions demanding elective double stenting.

Flow chart 12.2: Elective double stenting

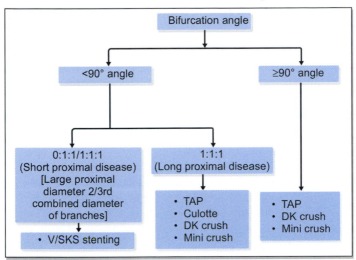

Abbreviations: TAP, T-stenting and small protrusion; DK crush, double-kissing crush

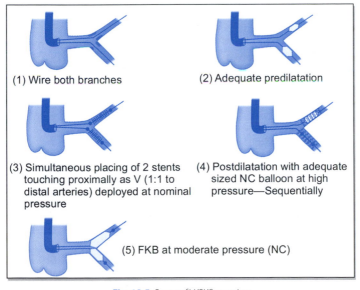

Fig. 12.5: Steps of V/SKS stenting
Abbreviations: NC, non-compliant; FKB, final kissing balloon

Individual Techniques

V stenting and simultaneous Kissing stenting (SKS): These techniques are of limited use now for the fear of difficult future intervention. Mainly recommended in LM situations where proximal artery is free of disease (Fig. 12.5).

Advantage: Both stents can be delivered and deployed together without losing access to any of the two branches.

Requirement:
- The size of the proximal vessel must be large (> 2/3rd of combined diameter of the daughter vessels).

- If the proximal vessel (e.g. LMCA) is short, free of disease, particularly in the time of emergency—V stenting is a very useful technique.
- Two stents in two daughter arteries should enter the mother vessel and touch each other forming a new carina. This entry into main branch should be around 2 mm in V stenting and ≥ 3 mm in SKS.
- The angle between the two daughter vessels should be < 90°.

Specific Issues in SKS

- Long-term outcome is not known
- Possible barotraumas in LMCA
- If there is a proximal dissection in LMCA, it is very difficult to treat and always there is a chance of directing the flow towards the stent.
- If there is a proximal restenosis one stent needs to be crushed. To enter side branch through 4 layers of stent is always challenging. Even in distal restenosis or disease distal to the stent, it is difficult to negotiate the wire upto the distal segment due to crisscross through the Stent struts.

Crush technique (Figs 12.6 and 12.7): Basic philosophy of the technique is crushing the SB stent by MB stent, so that the ostium of SB is never missed. Classical crush involves crushing ≥ 5 mm SB stent by MB stent leading to difficult crossing into SB and final kissing balloon inflation (FKI). The crush technique has evolved and is nowadays performed with less stent protrusion into MB (i.e. Mini crush/DK crush) and mandatory two FKI.

Specific Issues in Mini Crush and DK Crush

- Mini crush or DK crush both can be done in cases where the angle between the daughter vessel is ≥ 90°.

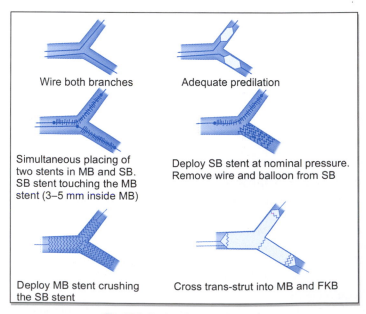

Wire both branches

Adequate predilation

Simultaneous placing of two stents in MB and SB. SB stent touching the MB stent (3–5 mm inside MB)

Deploy SB stent at nominal pressure. Remove wire and balloon from SB

Deploy MB stent crushing the SB stent

Cross trans-strut into MB and FKB

Fig. 12.6: Crush technique: Mini crush

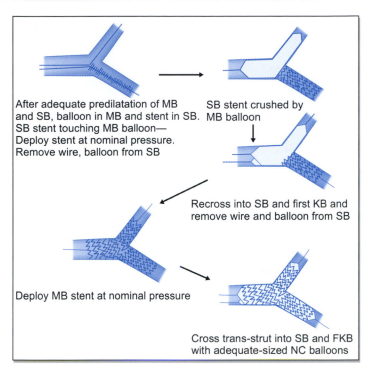

After adequate predilatation of MB and SB, balloon in MB and stent in SB. SB stent touching MB balloon—Deploy stent at nominal pressure. Remove wire, balloon from SB

SB stent crushed by MB balloon

Recross into SB and first KB and remove wire and balloon from SB

Deploy MB stent at nominal pressure

Cross trans-strut into SB and FKB with adequate-sized NC balloons

Fig. 12.7: Crush technique: DK Crush

- Both techniques involve minimal stent protrusion in MB making side branch entry after MB stenting easier.
- Two step FKI—firstly high pressure dilation of side branch by NC balloon after crossing trans-strut into SB and then FKI—opens the ostium of SB nicely and leads to proper apposition.

Culotte Stenting (Fig. 12.8)

Can be used in almost all true bifurcation lesions irrespective of bifurcation angle, where there is no major discrepancy in size between MB and SB. If the bifurcation angle is more than 90°, Culotte is not a preferred mode of stenting.

Specific issues in culotte stenting:
- Technically more challenging
- Stenting the SB first does not always guarantee against acute closure of MB.

T Stenting and protrusion (TAP technique) (Fig. 12.9): As the current consensus is to consider provisional stenting as the default strategy for most bifurcations, in up to 30% of cases treated with provisional stenting require cross over to 2-stent strategy due to flow compromise in the SB. T stenting and small protrusion (TAP) is a relatively new technique which is technically less challenging and ensures complete coverage of SB ostium and minimizes stent overlap. Unlike other strategies the TAP technique does not require recrossing of the stent to perform FKI.

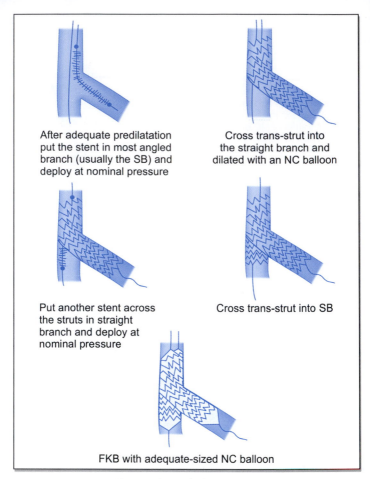

After adequate predilatation put the stent in most angled branch (usually the SB) and deploy at nominal pressure

Cross trans-strut into the straight branch and dilated with an NC balloon

Put another stent across the struts in straight branch and deploy at nominal pressure

Cross trans-strut into SB

FKB with adequate-sized NC balloon

Fig. 12.8: Steps of culotte stenting

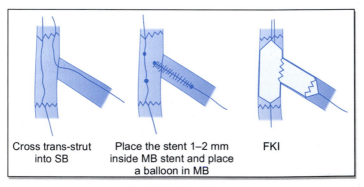

Cross trans-strut into SB

Place the stent 1–2 mm inside MB stent and place a balloon in MB

FKI

Fig. 12.9: TAP technique

Methods:
- Steps like provisional stenting
- After crossing the SB through the MB stent strut 2nd stent is advanced in the SB in a way to minimally protrude (1 or 2 mm) into the MB where a stent has already been implanted.

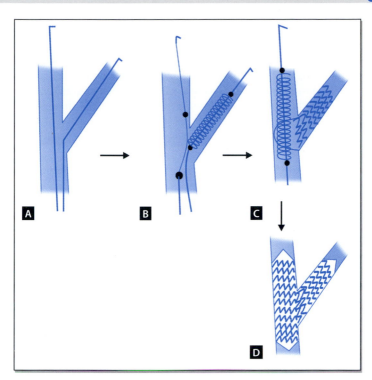

Figs 12.10A to D: Modified flower petal technique. (A) Wiring both branches (adequate pre-dilatation); (B) Balloon through the last strut of the SB stent assembly placed; (C) MB stent; (D) Kissing balloon

- A balloon is advanced into the MB
- SB stent is deployed as usual (12 atm or more) and MB balloon is simultaneously inflated at 12 atmosphere pressure or more.
- Both balloons are deflated and removed.

Specific issues: TAP is a good technique when the angle between the daughter vessels is ≤ 90°.

Modified flower petal technique: Despite the widespread applications of DES, restenosis of the ostium of the SB is still unresolved, regardless of the variety of bifurcation stenting methods—The main reason is incomplete coverage of the SB ostium (T-stenting) or inadequate final opening of the ostium (as in most crush stenting where FKB is often difficult and inadequate due to multiple layer of stents).

A new technique has been proposed by Kinoshito and modified by Cayli called Flower petal technique which ensues complete coverage of the ostium with minimal metal load.

The technique is described in Figures 12.10A to D.

Comments:
- The technique is complex
- Intertwining of the guidewires may be a problem
- Stent dislodgement may take place
- Not suitable for tortuous lesions
- Not an ideal technique in wider angle bifurcation.

Bifurcation Stenting: Summary

In most of the cases of bifurcation stenosis single stent strategy for MB and provisional stenting of SB is an effective strategy. Elective double stenting should be tried in specific indications and it is mandatory to finish the procedure with two step final kissing balloon inflation.

The operator should resist temptation to improve angiographic appearance because focal restenosis at the SB is very frequently clinically silent, and also many ostially narrow, jailed SBs are not functionally significant (Fractional Flow Reserve > 0.8).

Ostial Lesions

Ostial disease is traditionally defined as a lesion arising within 3 mm of the vessel origin. It may be classified by location as aorto-ostial and branch-ostial.

Aorto-ostial disease is more common in women and right coronary artery (RCA) ostium is involved more than left coronary artery (LCA) ostium. Like all other coronary artery lesions, etiology is mostly atherosclerotic. As the aorto-ostial part of the artery is almost an extension of aortic structure, the lesions in this part of the artery is more fibrotic, calcified, relatively rigid, prone to recoil, dissection and vessel closure.

There are certain problems which are inherent to ostial diseases which influence the strategy of PCI. They are as follows:

1. **Exclusion of coronary spasm:** Engagement of catheters at the aorto-ostial sites may provoke spasm and give a false impression of severe ostial disease. A high index of suspicion is required, especially, if no significant coronary plaque is evident elsewhere. Appropriate measures to avoid or detect coronary spasm include the use of intra-coronary nitrates, smaller diameter catheters, nonselective contrast injection into the appropriate coronary sinus.

2. **Ostial LAD stenosis:** A decision has to be taken as a strategy at the outset, whether precise positioning of the stent at the ostium should be attempted or whether stenting across left circumflex coronary artery (LCX) into left main coronary artery (LMCA) is preferable. In this respect following characteristics help in decision making.
   a. The presence or absence of an ostial 'nub' or stump to facilitate proximal positioning.
   b. The angle of bifurcation with LCX—Angles <75° are associated with greater difficulty in stent positioning and increased risk of plaque shift (Figs 12.11A and B).
   c. The presence of significant plaque in distal LMCA or LCX ostium which may dictate an alternate strategy.
   d. The presence of heavy calcification which may impair visualization and stent positioning, limit stent expansion—requiring plaque modification and debulking.
   e. Discrepancy between the size of LAD and LMCA, can change the strategy of stenting.

3. **Side branch ostial stenosis**: Always consider risk and benefit for the procedure and in most of the cases medical therapy is favored.

4. **Ostial stenosis following previous bifurcation PCI:** Restenosis at the ostium of a side branch following a previous bifurcation procedure is not infrequent. Options include avoidance of further PCI, particularly when the affected vessel is a branch artery.

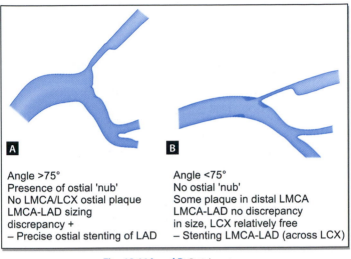

Angle >75°
Presence of ostial 'nub'
No LMCA/LCX ostial plaque
LMCA-LAD sizing
discrepancy +
– Precise ostial stenting of LAD

Angle <75°
No ostial 'nub'
Some plaque in distal LMCA
LMCA-LAD no discrepancy
in size, LCX relatively free
– Stenting LMCA-LAD (across LCX)

Figs 12.11A and B: Ostial anatomy

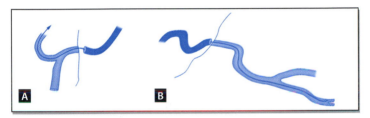

Figs 12.12A and B: Buddy Wires. (A) Buddy wire to stabilize guide catheter;
(B) Extra-support wire to stabilize guide catheter

Methods

Guide catheters: Guide catheter selection is important for aorto-ostial disease because of fear of dissection of the ostium. Less aggressive catheters like Judkins should be chosen for going in or out of the ostium during stent manipulation.

Side-hole catheters are not recommended as the warning sign of pressure damping from catheter wedging and flow compromise is obscured.

Guidewires: Standard work-horse wires are sufficient to finish the job perfectly. A few small tricks are sometimes necessary to overcome problems, for example:

1. A buddy wire in one of the early branches may sometimes be required to stabilize the guide catheter (Figs 12.12A and B).
2. In severe aorto-ostial disease it is advisable to preload the wire in the guide before vessel intubation to facilitate rapid wiring and catheter disengagement, if necessary.
3. An extra-support wire sometimes may be required if guide catheter's position in ascending aorta is precious (as may be the case for aorto-coronary bypass graft with superior origin).

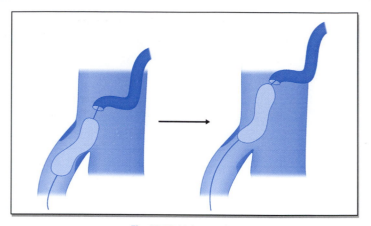

Fig. 12.13: Melon seeding

Preparation of bed before stenting: Lesion preparation before stenting is essential due to rigidity of the ostial lesions which is observed more often than not. For aorto-ostial lesion due to presence of high amount elastic fibers, balloons frequently slip out (Melon seeding, Fig. 12.13)—which may be prevented by following measures.

Prevention of Melon seeding:
1. Use another wire as a buddy wire and try focused force angioplasty
2. Use cutting balloon/Scoring balloon/Angiosculpt to open the lesion
3. Rotational atherectomy in severely calcified lesions (rail track calcification in fluoroscopy).

Positioning of the stent:
Ostial PCI requires very precise stent positioning to obtain full lesion coverage, yet avoid unnecessary proximal extension which may result in obstruction of major vessels or excessive overhang into the aorta. It is necessary to reiterate that the stent is within the radioactive markers on the stent balloon and thus the proximal marker must be positioned proximal to the ostium in any ostial lesion.

Methods of proper positioning:
Visualization of the ostial position properly is the key of success. Different angulated angiographic views are to be tried to choose the right one which exposes the ostium properly and widely separates the branches and reveal the angle in case of branch ostial lesion. Always remember that the ideal angle is at least > 75° (Table 12.1).

If the angle is < 75°, then it is impossible to place the stent in side branch ostium with proper coverage without having stent impingement of the main branch (Fig. 12.14).

Positioning of stent in aorto-ostial lesion: Stenting of aorto-ostial lesion requires guide catheter disengagement, yet still allowing visualization and avoiding prolapse of the stent, wire into aorta. Tricks are:
1. After positioning the stent, a small forward push on guidewire can disengage guide catheter.
2. With the proximal stent marker outside the guide but fully within the vessel, tighten the T-B connector and retract guide and stent as a single unit along with the wire (Fig. 12.15).

Table 12.1: Angiographic views for different ostial lesions

Vessel with ostial lesion	Suggested views
LMS	AP cranial/AP
RCA	LAO/LAO caudal
LAD	LAO caudal/AP caudal (Varying LAO and caudal angles)*
LCX	LAO caudal (Varying LAO and caudal angles)*
Bypass graft	LAO/lateral ± caudal for RCA grafts
	RAO view for LCA grafts (least foreshortened)

*[From Yahoo (LAO 90°, caudal 32°) to shallow (LAO 10–15°, caudal 20–40°)]

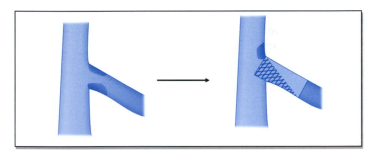

Fig. 12.14: Impingement (plaque shift + stent protrusion)

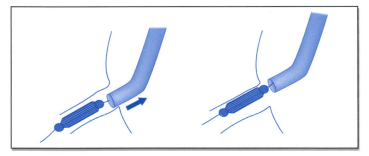

Fig. 12.15: Ostial stent positioning

Excessive respiratory/cardiac motion:
Particularly problematic with ostial LAD stenting where oscillation of the LAD stent increases the risk of inaccurate placement.

Shallow respiration and period of apnea just before stent placement and inflation for excessive respiratory movement.

Excessive cardiac motion is especially most problematic for ostial LAD.

Two specialized stent positioning techniques are described for proper positioning.

1. **Stent drawback technique:** See Figure 12.16

2. **Szabo technique:** See Figure 12.17

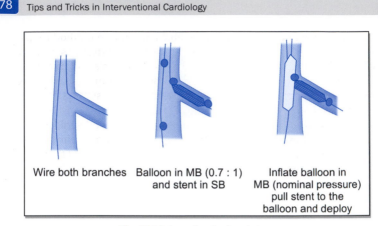

Wire both branches

Balloon in MB (0.7 : 1) and stent in SB

Inflate balloon in MB (nominal pressure) pull stent to the balloon and deploy

Fig. 12.16: Stent drawback technique

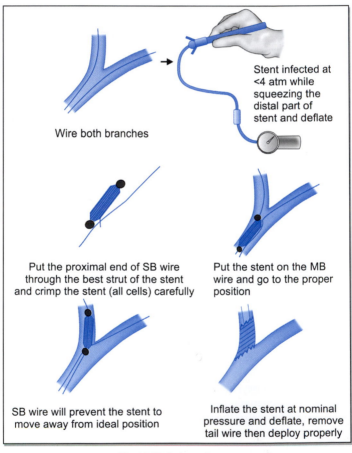

Wire both branches

Stent infected at <4 atm while squeezing the distal part of stent and deflate

Put the proximal end of SB wire through the best strut of the stent and crimp the stent (all cells) carefully

Put the stent on the MB wire and go to the proper position

SB wire will prevent the stent to move away from ideal position

Inflate the stent at nominal pressure and deflate, remove tail wire then deploy properly

Fig. 12.17: Szabo technique

In 2005, Szabo reported a method of using two guidewires to enable optimal coverage of the ostium. The guidewires are placed in MB and SB or in the aorta if an aorto-ostial lesion is being treated. The steps are described in Figure 12.17. Szabo technique shows angiographically perfect positioning of the stent. A recent analysis (Vaquerizo) suggests that Szabo technique is not a predictable and precise method to use for implanting a stent at the ostium of a coronary artery. As a result of data from IVUS, angiographic analysis of restenosis and micro CT bench testing, it may be concluded that Szabo technique is a complex technique with relatively low immediate angiographic success (88.5%). When compared to other recent simpler techniques, mid-term results appeared to be worse. Despite of limitations, there is still a role for the Szabo technique in ostial stent placement and many of its limitations can be overtaken by proper predilatation, proper crimping of the stent, avoiding intertwining of the two guidewires and final post dilatation with a high pressure balloon.

Precautions for Szabo technique:
1. 7F Guide catheter is advisable to minimize stent friction
2. Proper preparation of the bed (the lesion) before stenting (if required plaque modification/debulking) for proper movement of the stent.
3. Crimp the stent properly after putting tail wire otherwise stent may get dislodged.
4. Be careful about intertwining of the wire, if suspect intertwining pull back the stent system and try to re-cross without twisting.
5. Always be careful not to damage the balloon during putting the tail wire through the last strut of the stent.
6. Do not use polymer coated wire as an anchor wire.

Floating-stent technique: It consists of implanting a DES in the proximal LAD to partially cover the origin of LCX without further planned intervention (Fig. 12.18).

We know that a shallow angle between LAD and LCX is predictive of LCX ostium impairment after stenting with a cut-off of 70°. Sometimes

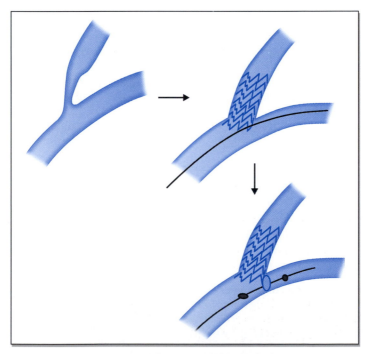

Fig. 12.18: Floating-stent technique

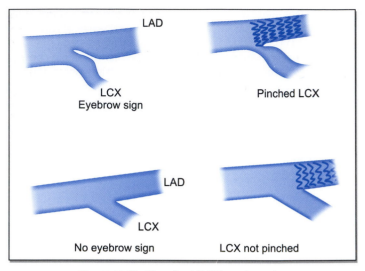

Fig. 12.19: Pinching of ostial LCX in eyebrow sign

the angles are not clearly perceived in angiography due to overlapping or foreshortening of the proximal part of the branches. Medina et al. proposed this floating stent technique after IVUS examination of LAD to LMCA, observing that those with a specific feature called 'eye brow sign' in longitudinal reconstruction of IVUS image are prone to develop LCX ostial impairment (Fig. 12.19).

Floating stent technique can be used if IVUS shows:
- No eyebrow signs
- LAD plaque mainly located at the ostium without involving distal LMCA
- LCX ostium does not show any significant plaque accumulation
  According to the authors in situations where the lesion is suitable for floating stent technique no compromise of the LCX ostium (takes place), at all there is a compromise that is usually mild and can be easily managed by passing a guidewire through the distal cell covering LCX ostium and a low atmosphere balloon dilatation, is all that if necessary to reposition the carina. Kissing balloon is not advisable to avoid barotraumas in the distal LMCA, which is not protected by the stent.

Percutaneous Coronary Intervention in a Tortuous Artery

Coronary tortuosity can be defined when an artery is having more than 3 bends (defined as $\geq 45^0$ change in vessel direction) along main trunk present both in systole and diastole (Fig. 12.20). Female gender and hypertension are most common associates.

Problems of tortuous artery intervention:
1. Difficulty in wiring the vessel
2. Pseudolesions (concertina effect)
3. Difficulty in tracking the device (stents, balloons)

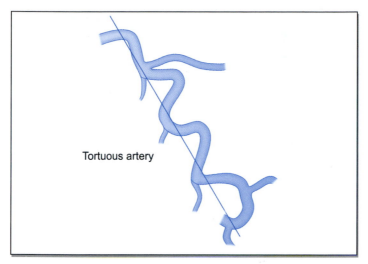

Fig. 12.20: PCI in tortuous artery

Tips and tricks: It is always difficult to cross the lesions in a tortuous artery. So following things should be planned before hand:

1. Good guide catheter back-up
   - Using passive support catheter OR
   - Using active guide catheter for
   a. Deep throttling (using a 5F/6F with/without anchor balloon)
   b. Mother and child
   c. Guide-liner catheter
2. Using hydrophilic wire to cross and then using a buddy wire (exchanging with extra support on a microcatheter).

Extra-support wires—Ironman (Abbott Vascular), Grand slam (Asahi), Platinum Plus (Boston Scientific) can make the artery straight and make device tracking easier. Sometimes two buddy wires are used for better tracking. Extra-support wires may cause vasoconstriction particularly at the bends producing pseudolesions or concertina. Sometimes these pseudolesions pose difficulty in choosing the stent length.

Trouble shooting
- Fix the lesion length before putting the extra-support wire
- Put the stent distally to cross the original lesion
- If you have any doubt about pseudolesion exchange extra-support wire on a microcatheter give NTG/NIKORANDIL intracoronary, which can abolish concertina.

Difficulty in Stent Tracking

When a stent fails to cross a tortuous angulated lesion site, the basic principles of stent technique should be invoked—maximize guide catheter support, optimize predilatation of the stenosis, utilize a stiffer and use a more flexible, shorter or lower profile stent system. Further use of specific tricks is often helpful (Table 12.2).

Occasionally, however despite the application of standard and non-standard techniques, a situation is encountered where stent passage appears impossible.

Table 12.2: Techniques useful for stent delivery in tortuous anatomy

	Strategy	Possible mechanism
Guide	Deep seating	Better guide support
	Guide with different curve or Amplatz guide	Optimal coaxial support
	Larger caliber guide	More support
	Smaller caliber guide	Deep seating
Guidewire	Iron man, platinum plus or 0.018 wire	More support
	Less support wire	More flexible
	Bent wire	Deviates local wire bias
	Superstiff buddy wire	Straightens tortuosity
Stent	Bent stent	Aligns stent with tortuosity
	Bubble stent	Improves trackability
	Shorter stent	Better chance at crossing sharp angles
Vessel	Accept angioplasty result	No stent needed
	Optimize predilatation or debulk plaque	Less luminal obstruction

Table 12.3: Special techniques for stent delivery in tortuous lesions

- Buddy wire and wires (Fig. 12.21)
- Jailed buddy wire (Fig. 12.22)
- Anchor balloon (Fig. 12.23)
- Balloon deflation technique (Fig. 12.24)
- Forward pressure with partial stent—balloon inflation

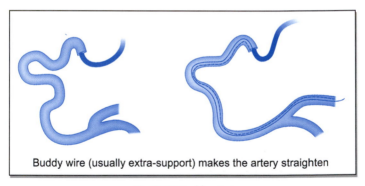

Buddy wire (usually extra-support) makes the artery straighten

Fig. 12.21: Buddy wires

Marked tortuosity and vessel angulations remain a challenge for stent delivery despite the advances in stent delivery systems and trackability of newer stents. Some techniques to deal with this scenario may not be applicable in certain situations and some may be potentially risky in others while one can anticipate difficulties on viewing the coronary anatomy. It is not possible to predict which bend will create problem in the passage of the stents. Rigid and calcified vessels are notorious for such behavior. Sharp angulations of the native coronary arteries caused by the hook-up of the bypass graft is also resistant to unimpeded passage of the stents (Table 12.3).

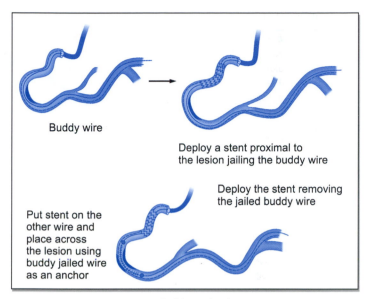

Fig. 12.22: Buddy-in-jail technique

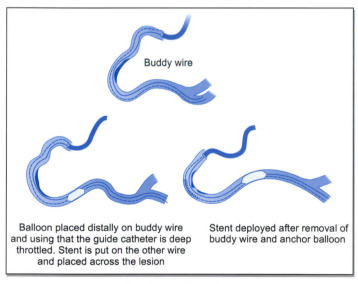

Fig. 12.23: Anchor balloon

A large diameter (at least 7 Fr) guide catheter should be used, to allow simultaneous handling of the buddy wire and the wire delivering stent or other equipment.

Buddy-in-jail Technique (Fig. 12.22)

Two wires are advanced distal to the target lesion, one buddy wire, and one main wire which will be utilized for delivery of stent. A stent is deployed along the main wire, just proximal to the target lesion, and thus jailing the buddy wire to the wall of the artery. Now another stent

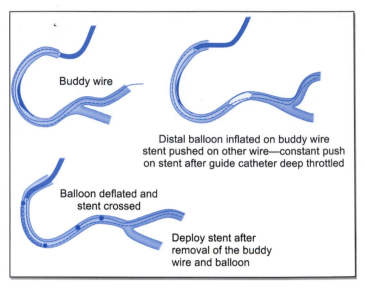

Buddy wire

Distal balloon inflated on buddy wire
stent pushed on other wire—constant push
on stent after guide catheter deep throttled

Balloon deflated and
stent crossed

Deploy stent after
removal of the buddy
wire and balloon

Fig. 12.24: Balloon deflation technique

is put on the other wire and the lesion is crossed easily, with the the jailed buddy wire as an anchor. The stent advancement is easier and is facilitated by the presence of a 'buddy' wire (better traction and deep throttling of the guide catheter). The stent is deployed across the lesion, while removing the jailed buddy wire.

Anchor Balloon Technique (Fig. 12.23)

Two wires are advanced distal to the target lesion to enable utilization of the trapping balloon and the equipment in need of delivery, usually a stent. The distal trapping balloon is advanced distally beyond the target lesion and inflated usually at 10–12 atm. Either a compliant or noncompliant balloon can be utilized, although compliant balloons are more deliverable through tortuous and calcified coronary artery segments. Now, as the buddy wire is anchored with balloon, the guide catheter can be deep throttled over it. Finally, the stent is advanced toward the target lesion. Once the stent reaches the target lesion, the distal balloon is deflated and withdrawn, along with the buddy wire, and stent is deployed.

Balloon Deflation Technique (Fig. 12.24)

Two wires are advanced distal to the target lesion to enable utilization of the trapping balloon and the equipment in need of delivery, usually a stent. Now, a balloon is delivered distally and inflated at a normal pressure to allow deep throttling of the guide catheter. With better stability of deep throttled guide catheter, finally, the stent is advanced toward the target lesion. Once the stent reaches the distal anchor balloon and the target lesion, the distal balloon is deflated and withdrawn, along with a continuous forward pressure on the stent and suddenly the stent crosses the lesion. The buddy wire along with deflated balloon is removed and stent is deployed.

Forward pressure with partial stent-balloon inflation:
After adequate predilatation, a highly trackable and flexible stent is advanced into the vessel over a stiff wire as far as it will go. Firm forward pressure is then applied on the stent-balloon at the loosened hemostatic valve such that some of the catheter tubing is advanced into the port while no forward progress is seen at the stent end. This maintains a constant forward pressure. The stent-balloon is gently inflated to 2–3 atm. The stretch of the minimally inflated balloon straightens the impending segment. The forward pressure maintained on the balloon directs the stent in the required direction. The nesting of the stent on the balloon prevents the stent from slipping off the balloon at low pressure inflation. When the stent advances to the target site—it is fully deployed at recommended pressures.

Calcified Lesions

Vascular calcification is hydroxyapatite crystal deposit within the intima or less frequently in the media resulting from passive physicochemical and active cellular processes. Coronary artery lesions are frequently calcified, yet the low sensitivity of angiography often leaves them undetected. Thus compared to IVUS, coronary angiography can detect 25% of one quadrant calcium (< 90°), 50% of two quadrant and 60% of three quadrant and 85% of four quadrant calcium lesions. Calcified lesions may be bad or good news. Calcium gives stability of the lesion and prevents positive remodeling, whereas heavily calcified lesions are rigid and therefore more difficult to dilate. High pressure dilatation may lead to vessel perforation and dissection and in heavily calcified lesions, there is always a fear of stent under expansion and malapposition leading to stent thrombosis. Low grade proximal (<50%) calcified lesions may complicate access to more distal severe lesions (culprit), where reaching the lesion with balloon/stent sometime becomes extremely difficult.

How you plan to do a calcified lesion?
- If angiography demonstrates rail-track calcification (> 10 mm in length) or severe calcification (equivalent to > 180° arc of calcification in superficial layers by IVUS)–**Rotablation**
- Rail-track calcification (<10 mm in length) Moderate calcification (90–180° arc of calcification in the superficial layers of plaque by IVUS)–**Rota/Cutting balloon/Angiosculpt**
- Undilatable lesion (Balloon not fully inflated @ 10 atm) or mild calcification—**Use IVUS before to confirm before selecting the device and cutting balloon/Angiosculpt/Scoring balloon.**

Rotablation: Tips and Tricks

Rotational atherectomy (RA) or Rotablator was developed to remove calcified or fibrotic plaque by pulverizing it to micro-particles by a rotating diamond coated mandrel in 1988 by David Auth. The device preferentially ablates hard, calcific atherosclerotic plaque but does not affect the normal elastic tissue in the same way, a razor shaves the beard without cutting the skin.

Rotational atherectomy (RA) acts by orthogonal displacement of friction functions. Friction develops in a longitudinal direction between the guidewire and the device, in RA high speed rotation changes the friction vector to a circumferential rotation which allows burr advancement through tight tortuous vessels and lesions.

Plaque Modification versus Debulking

Rotational atherectomy as a procedure went out of favor following trials showing high restenosis rate, but it has undergone a resurgence of interest mainly due to:

- More and more referral to cardiac intervention of elderly patients with heavily calcified coronary arteries
- Expansion of PCI indications to more challenging anatomic subsets as a consequence of the improved restenosis rate following drug-eluting stent (DES).

Over the years, the major adverse cardiac events (MACE) rate of rotational atherectomy has been reduced significantly. Khattab et al. have compared the outcomes between drug-eluting and bare metal stents following rotational atherectomy in calcified lesions. They have reported significant reduction in restenosis rates with the use of DES (7.4% vs 35.2%) in small group of patients.

Unlike balloon dilatation that results in the displacement of the atherosclerotic plaque with multiple intimal tears, rotational atherectomy is based on the principle of differential cutting that allows for physical removal of inelastic atherosclerotic material while rendering the inner lumen surface smooth. Although, plaque reduction by pulverization of the atherosclerotic material into microparticles has remained its central paradigm, the conceptual framework has shifted from debulking to plaque modification prior to stent implantation. In 2016, Sakakura et al. (Circulation: Cardiovascular Intervention, 2016) showed that in nation-wide registry of PCI, rotational atherectomy (RA) was 3.2% in 2014 and 2015 and the combined incidence of major complications defined as in-hospital death, cardiac tamponade and emergent surgery was 1.31%, which was similar to overall registry population.

Probably, these data could be explained by more frequent use of optimal RA technique, which is tailored to serve as a complication avoidance strategy (Table 12.4).

Brief Description of the Equipment

The rotational atherectomy (RA) system includes the burr, Rota wire, console and nitrogen tank.

The console: The console is the office of Rotablator system, it is connected to advancer, turbine and foot pedal and controls total event. The features are described in Figure 12.25.

Foot pedal: The foot pedal is used as an on/off control for the advancer gas turbine. The foot pedal is also fitted with a valve which vents any compress gas in the foot-pedal hose when the pedal is released permitting rapid stopping of the burr. Dynaglide button located on the right side of the foot pedal housing is used as on/off control for the dynaglide mode of operation. When dynaglide is on, the green 'Dynaglide' light is illuminated on the console front panel (dynaglide allows low rotation at 60,000 to 90,000 rpm) (Fig. 12.26).

Table 12.4: Contemporary rotational atherectomy

Arterial access	Radial (6–7 F) Femoral (7F)
Guiding catheter	Single curve with strong support
Burr size	Small burrs (usually 1.25 to 1.5) always less than 0.6
Ablation speed	• 140000 to 150000 rpm based on the finding that burr speed is linearly associated with platelet aggregation • Avoidance of deceleration > 5000 rpm for cumulative > 5 sec, because the loss in speed was associated with periprocedural myocardial infarction (MI) and restenosis. • Burr advancement using pecking motion in short ablative runs of 15 to 20 sec. to avoid vessel injury and burr entrapment
Avoiding TPM routinely atropine may be used instead	
Continuous intracoronary flushing with NTG/Heparin Verapamil and Nikorandil or adenosine to prevent no re-flow	

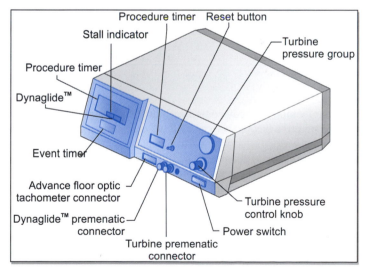

Fig. 12.25: Rota console

Nitrogen/air cylinder: To be attached at the back of the console and pressure adjusted so that pneumatic pressure becomes adequate for proper functioning of the burr.

The Burr and Advancer (Rota link Plus): The new system of Rota link plus combines burr and advancer together. The diamond-coated burr

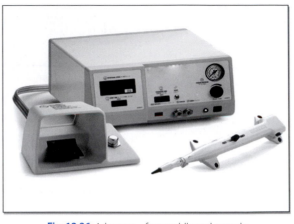

Fig. 12.26: Advancer—foot paddle and console

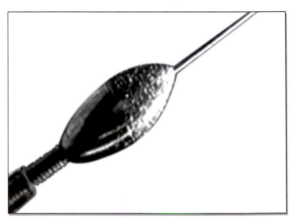

Fig. 12.27: Rota burr

consists of a tapered body coated with fine diamond chips. The burr is connected to a flexible helical shaft which has a central lumen that permits passage of the guidewire. The advancer acts as a support for the air turbine and as a guide for the sliding elements which control burr extension. The air turbine uses compressed gas to generate the high rotational speed necessary for ablation. Components are described in Figures 12.27 and 12.28.

Other Hardwares

Guide catheter: Coaxiality of guide catheter is extremely important in RA. Coaxiality will reduce the tension or pull required on the guidewire when advancing the burr. Significant support or deep intubation generally is not needed with this device since activation of the burr provides orthogonal displacement of friction which will reduce the drag to ease the passage of the burr through the vessel. Also coaxiality will provide the orientation of the guidewire centrally, therefore, overriding guidewire bias (divergence from central axis of the vessel) (Fig. 12.29).

Guide catheter inner diameter should be 0.004″, larger than the largest burr used (Table 12.5).

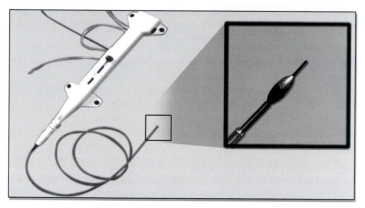

Fig. 12.28: Burr with Advancer

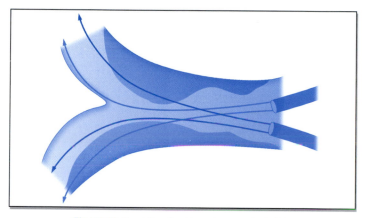

Fig. 12.29: Coaxiality of guide catheter and wire bias

Table 12.5: Relationship of burr size and guide catheter size

Burr size	In inches	Guide catheter
1.25 mm	0.049	6F
1.50 mm	0.059	6F
1.75 mm	0.069	7F
2 mm	0.079	7F
2.15 mm	0.085	8F
2.25 mm	0.089	8F
2.38 mm	0.094	9F
2.50 mm	0.098	9F

Guidewire: The two unique guidewires are used for directing the burr are the Rota floppy and Rota extra-support guidewires. The length of the wire is 330 mm and the body of the wire is 0.009 inches. The maximum tip diameter is 0.014 inch. The Rota floppy guidewire has a long-tapered shaft that is designed for greater flexibility and to minimize unfavorable guidewire bias. The extra-support guidewire has a short, tapered shaft that maximizes straightening of the vessel and provides extra support

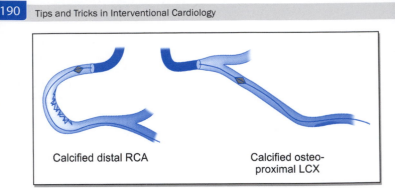

Calcified distal RCA

Calcified osteo-
proximal LCX

Fig. 12.30: Rota extra-support wire

during advancement of the burr into the lesions. In more than 90% cases, Rota floppy wire is enough to complete the procedure. Extra-support wires are required in heavily calcified proximal lesions or in distal lesions (Fig. 12.30).

The Cocktail (Rota flush): It is used to cool down heat generated during ablation and to prevent spasm of the artery. The flow should be 6–8 mL/30 sec during ablation. The flush contains:

Rota flush:
• 0.9 normal saline—500 mL
• Nitroglycerin—5 mg
• Heparin—1000 units
• Verapamil—5 mg

This should be contained in a plastic bag with pressure gauge to push water in required flow. Never operate the Rotablator advancer without saline infusion on.

Pre-procedure test: DRAW

Drip	Saline drip from bottom of advancer and catheter
Rotate	Burr is rotating and RPMs are stable
Advancer	Free movement of advancer knob
Wire	Wire is visible, brake is functioning (observe the wire and brake behind the advancer, and look for stability of the wire while foot pedal is on for burr rotation, i.e. no spinning of the wire itself)

Steps of Rotablation

• Place Rota guidewire across the lesion. Two important things to remember:
  1. Rota wires are less torquable, so it is better to cross the lesion with a general guidewire and exchange it with a Rota guidewire on a microcatheter.
  2. Rota wires should be handled carefully, if the wire gets kinked, it should be replaced before further procedure.
• Put the burr on the wire like an over the wire balloon and test the rotation before entering 'Y' connector. The rotation should be kept between 1,40,000 to 1,60,000 rpm.

- 'Y' connector should not be very tight so that free movement of burr becomes possible, otherwise there may be stalking of burr or damage of drive shaft.

  The experimental study revealed that the reduction of burr speed to the minimal approved level (1,40,000 rpm) much reduced platelet aggregation due to heat generation. This low speed treatment may be beneficial for avoiding slow flow and no-reflow which often complicated the treatment of lesions with highly complex morphology, especially in long lesion, but it takes longer ablation time and needs more refined hands.
- Check the Cocktail flow
- Check the advancer knob and lock it 2–3 cm forward before advancing burr into guide catheter
- Advance the burr forward while holding the wire
- Place the burr 2–3 cm ahead of the lesion, it is the platform. Then, the advancer knob is moved back slightly to release the tension of the burr shaft
- Put the wire clip torquer on the wire behind the advancer and start ablation
- Do not push the Rotablator burr into the lesion, use 'Pecking' technique (Pecking technique is used, where the burr is moved forward and backward to the lesion, avoiding crossing the entire lesion during initial passage. Pecking motion prevents 'trenching' into arterial wall, allows wire to reposition as vessel compliance changes with debulking)
- Do not allow ablation more than 15 seconds. Stop in the platform and allow Rotaflush to flow, to prevent slow flow, bradycardia and hypotension
- If there is hypotension start inotropes
- During ablation excessive deceleration (more than 5,000 rpm) must be avoided, because it results in improper ablation, increases the risk of vessel injury, large particle formation and ischemic complications related to excessive heat generation.

Other cautions in ablating technique:
- Avoid rapid movement, Dottering force
- Avoid stopping or starting the burr in the lesion
- Avoid stopping the burr distal to lesion
- Avoid adjusting RPM during ablation
- Avoid the burr to remain in one location while rotating at high speed
- Avoid burring in the guide catheter
- Finish with one polishing run.

Other issues:
- Prophylactic temporary pacemaker (especially for right coronary and left circumflex arteries)
- GP IIb/IIIa inhibitors during rotablation (operator's choice).

Complications (Table 12.6):
'An ounce of prevention is worth a pound of care': Benjamin Franklyn
- Slow flow/no reflow
- Perforation

Table 12.6: Complication management and prevention

	Techniques to be avoided	Strategy for resolution
Slow flow	Small burrs and low speed Be patient between runs	Optimization of BP, if low Use of IC nitrates, sodium nitroprusside, Adenosine Use flush cocktail
Dissection	Avoid cases with excessive tortuosity	Avoid further ablation, if dissection is identified Dissection management
Perforation	Commonly related to poor technique (oversizing burr, too angulated lesion/ artery, inappropriate speed)	Standard therapy for perforation
Burr entrapment	Rare complication usually avoided with careful case selection and good technique	Controlled push and pull of shaft Position 2nd wire for balloon placement Cautious deep intubation with mother and child catheter for more support surgery

- *Advancer stops:*
  - Check all connections
  - Check air source—make sure it is on and delivering 90–110 psi
  - Likely a lack of saline allowed heating of the system
  - New advancer needed, if no saline drip through advancer
- *Stall light lights up:*
  As a safety measure, the system automatically stalls when there is >15,000 rpm drop for a ½ second or more. In that situation.
  - Ensure the burr is not lodged
  - Pull back and re-platform proximal to the lesion
  - Ensure all connections are secure
  - Ensure air supply
  - Ensure saline flow
- *Stuck rotablator:* The nightmare, reported incidence 0.4%
  Stuck Rotablator burr may occur due to two reasons:
  1. A small burr can be advanced beyond a heavily calcified plaque before superficial ablation, especially when the burr is pushed firmly at high rotational speed. In this situation, the ledge of calcium proximal to the burr may prevent burr withdrawal. This phenomenon was named 'Kokesi' after the Japanese doll.
  2. The burr can be entrapped within a severely calcified long lesion especially angulated and concomitant coronary spasm. When a large burr was pushing vigorously against such lesion without sufficient pecking motion, the rotational speed may decrease significantly and burr entrapment may occur.

Troubleshooting: See Flow chart 12.3

Flow chart 12.3: Troubleshooting of stuck rota burr

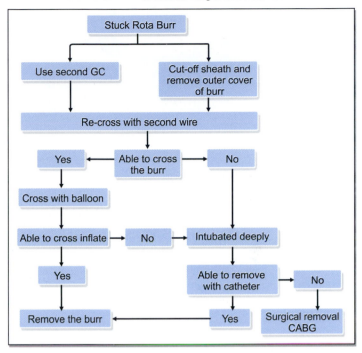

Chronic Total Occlusion (The Antegrade Way)

'The success of chronic total occlusion-percutaneous coronary invervention (CTO-PCI) is not only influenced by operator skill but also the operator's knowledge of devices and procedure.'

Chronic total occlusion is defined as a complete interruption of an antegrade blood flow (TIMI-0) as assessed by coronary angiography, despite vigorous injection, with an estimated occlusion duration of more than three months. The threshold of three months is directly related to the histological changes (fibrous tissue, more calcium, neo-channels, negative remodeling).

Prevalence: Approximately, one-third of patients with known or suspected coronary artery disease undergoing coronary angiogram present with CTO of at least one coronary vessel and 42–68% of the patients having CTO gives a history of prior myocardial infarction.

Anatomy and histopathology: CTOs most often arises from thrombotic occlusion, followed by thrombus organization and tissue aging. When there is a thrombotic occlusion of an artery, gradually thrombus becomes organized and gets replaced by collagen rich fibrous tissue, smooth muscle cells, intracellular and extracellular lipids and calcium. The collagen tissues are particularly dense at the proximal and distal ends of the lesion (proximal more than distal), and forms cap-like structure. At the ends between the caps, there are variable tissues which form a column. Depending on the tissue characters the typical CTO may be classified as 'soft', 'hard' or 'mixed' types (Fig. 12.31).

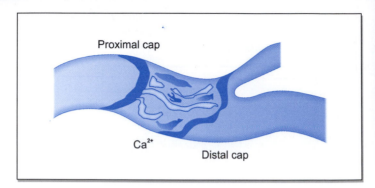

Fig. 12.31: Anatomy of CTO

Soft plaques consists of cholesterol laden cells and foam cells with loose fibrous tissue and neovascular channel, and is more frequent in younger occlusions (< 1 year).

Hard plaques are characterized by dense fibrous tissue and often contains large fibrocalcific regions without neovascular channels. These occlusions are more likely to deflect guidewires into subintimal area, creating dissection planes. Hard plaques are more prevalent with increasing age of CTO (> 1 year).

Microchannels: Intraluminal microchannels measuring 100–500 µm are commonly found in CTO. These channels facilitate the passage of guidewire. When these channels communicate with vasa vasorum in large amount, they are visible as bridging collaterals. In fact, visually detected microchannels are bad predictor for success, as they communicate with vasa-vasorum and cause extraluminal passage of wire.

Predictive Factors Related to Success or Failure of PCI for Chronic Total Occlusion (Fig. 12.32)

This is related to clinical, angiographic and clinical factors. It is a common mistake to restrict the number of projections during coronary angiography when a CTO is found. Multiple angiographic views and accurate frame by frame analysis of CTOs are necessary to evaluate the following angiographic characteristics, which are related to success or risk for complications of PCI.

Patient-related factors: CTO < 6 months is a factor which is correlated with better success, whereas CTO > 12 months is a stigma for difficult procedure or even failure (Table 12.7).

Success of percutaneous coronary intervention in chronic total occlusion has improved from 77% (in meta-analysis of 65 studies published between 2000 and 2011) to more than 94% between 2012 and 2015. This has been possible due to adoption of newer tools and techniques (hybrid approach).

How can the gap between what is achieved at most centers and what is achieved at experienced centers be bridged?

One answer is to increase dedicated CTO workers and another is to select proper cases that have a higher likelihood of success even with less experienced operators. Many angiographic and clinical scores have been

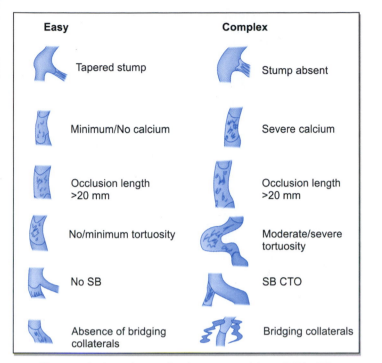

Easy	Complex
Tapered stump	Stump absent
Minimum/No calcium	Severe calcium
Occlusion length >20 mm	Occlusion length >20 mm
No/minimum tortuosity	Moderate/severe tortuosity
No SB	SB CTO
Absence of bridging collaterals	Bridging collaterals

Fig. 12.32: Predictive factors related to success or failure of PCI for CTO

Table 12.7: Complexity of chronic total occlusion (CTO)

Factors related to CTO	Level of PCI complexity	
	Easy	*Complex*
• Age of CTO	<6 months	>12 months
• Occlusion length	<20 mm	>20 mm
• Occlusion stump	Tapered	Blunt or absent
• Tortuosity at CTO	None/minimal	Moderate/severe
• Visibility of distal vessel	Good/excellent	Poor
• Ostial location	Yes	No
• CTO at proximal /mid-LCX	No	Yes
• Expected guide cath support	Good	Poor
• Previous attempts	No	Yes
• Expected patient tolerance	Good	Poor

developed to assist with patient selection for CTO-PCI. The most known score of CTO-PCI is the J-CTO (Multicenter CTO Registry in Japan) score, which was developed to predict successful guidewire crossing within 30 minutes. The J-CTO score has emerged as a useful prediction tool for antegrade success within defined procedure times (Table 12.8).

The North American algorithm to CTO-PCI was recently published. This algorithm was proposed as a decision tool (Brilakis ES, Kandzari DE. A percutaneous treatment algorithm for crossing coronary CTO. JACC Cardiovascular Intervention. 2012;5:367-79) (Flow chart 12.4)

Table 12.8: J-CTO score (Morino, Muramatsu, Katoh, JACC, Cardio Int. 2010)

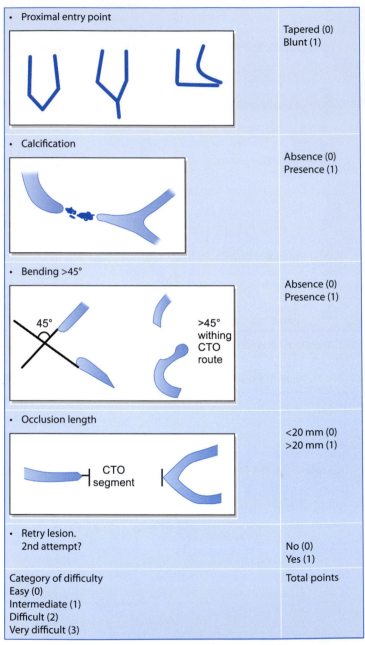

• Proximal entry point	Tapered (0) Blunt (1)
• Calcification	Absence (0) Presence (1)
• Bending >45°	Absence (0) Presence (1)
• Occlusion length	<20 mm (0) >20 mm (1)
• Retry lesion. 2nd attempt?	No (0) Yes (1)
Category of difficulty Easy (0) Intermediate (1) Difficult (2) Very difficult (3)	Total points

How should these scores be used to improve CTO-PCI outcomes?
- Outcomes could be improved by proper interpretation of Angiogram. At least 15 minutes of focused angiographic review is critical to understand the target.
- Plan according to the score assessed from coronary angiogram and select proper patient according to your ability (whether competent for hybrid procedures or antegrade only)
- Arrange your hardwares according to the plan.

Flow chart 12.4: A percutaneous treatment algorithm for crossing coronary CTO

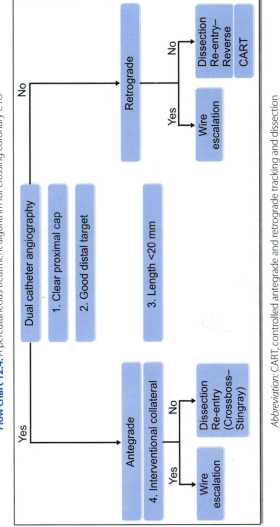

Abbreviation: CART, controlled antegrade and retrograde tracking and dissection

Steps of CTO Intervention—the Basics

- Planned procedure—not 'ad hoc'
- Assess diagnostic angiogram very carefully to assess
  1. The lost segment (calcification and tortuosity)
  2. Hardware required
  3. Collateral filled distal segment (bilateral angiography required if distal vessels filled—in all causes)
- Contrast volume calculation (according to eGFR and bodyweight)
- *Other factors:*
  1. Access issues
  2. If femoral (bilateral groin preparation for bilateral femoral access)
- Performing dual injection in nearly all cases
- Optimizing anticoagulation
- Applying various techniques to increase guide catheter support.

Hardwares for CTO Intervention

Guide Catheter

- Appropriate choice of guide catheter is the first step for success. Guide catheter should provide adequate support and coaxiality.
- Usually, a 7F catheter is a good general choice for antegrade complex. Chronic total occlusion A general rule for CTO is:

    For LAD: XB, XB LAD
         LCX: XB, Amplatz (L)
         RCA: Amplatz (L) 0.75/1, XB RCA

When proximal RCA disease is present use JR and avoid deep intubation. Sometimes guidewire support needs to be increased, e.g. in situations where CTO is crossed by guidewire but balloon is not crossing, in this situation following tricks may be helpful for increasing guide catheter support.

- Deep throttling of the guide catheter
- Side branch Anchor balloon technique
- GuideLiner, Guidezilla.

If there is tortuosity in the iliac or abdominal aorta take a long sheath to straighten the tortuosity as far as possible so that guide catheter support increases.

Microcatheters

Although standalone guidewire passage across a CTO can be achieved, microcatheter support is often required in complex CTOs. Micro-catheters are end-hole support catheter used to support the wire during CTO crossing, allow exchange of wires, help in parallel wiring without intertwining of the wires, also contrast injection and medications (GTN, Nicorandil) can be given through them in the distal arteries. Initially OTW balloons were used but they have been largely replaced by microcatheters.

A microcatheter can also straighten a curved and/or tortuous coronary artery proximal to the CTO and increase the guidewire torque so that it is close to 1:1.

In average CTO one can start the procedure with any microcatheter, e. g. Fine cross (Terumo), Valet (Volcano). Fine cross is very flexible and possesses the lowest crossing profile (1.7 Fr. Distal tip). It has a stainless

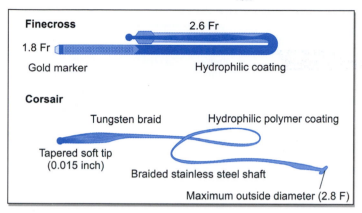

Fig. 12.33: Microcatheters

Table 12.9: Examples of microcatheters

1.	Corsair (Asahi)	2.5 F
2.	Progreat (Terumo)	2.4 F
3.	Tornus (Abbott/Asahi)	2.1 F/2.6 F
4.	Finecross (Terumo)	2 F
5.	Supercross (Vascular solutions)	2 F

steel braid (to enhance torquability) and a distal marker located 0.7 mm from the tip (Fig. 12.33 and Table 12.9).

Corsair microcatheter was developed (Asahi Intecc) as a channel dilator to facilitate retrograde PCI. The shaft is constructed with 8 thin wires wound with two large wires which facilitate torque transmission. The distal 60 cm is coated with the hydrophilic polymer to enhance crossability. It can be advanced by rotating counter clockwise and with associated forward push. Antegrade use of corsair is indicated whenever angulations and tortuosity of the coronary artery is encountered.

Tornus microcatheter (Asahi Intecc) is a novel OTW, flexible tapered metallic exchange catheter designed for complex and tight coronary lesions. It is 135 cm long and is available either as a 2.6 Fr or a more flexible 2.1 Fr. Version (Fig. 12.34). The catheter is advanced by counterclockwise rotation and pulled out with clockwise rotation. It is recommended to release torque energy after 20 rotations for the 2.6 F and 40 rotations for the 2.1 F catheter to avoid the risk of wire fracture. Tornus can be used in chronic total occlusion (CTO) and where wire has crossed the lesion but balloons are not crossing.

Guidewires for CTO

Basic Characteristics of a CTO Guidewire

Development of CTO guidewires by the industry and its evaluation had made CTO Intervention more predictable now than what was before. A CTO wire has some basic properties:

- *Type styles:* Core to tip designs, sometimes tapered.
- *Coils and covers:* Some favor increased radiopacity, joint-less coils for improved torque response, and polymer cover for

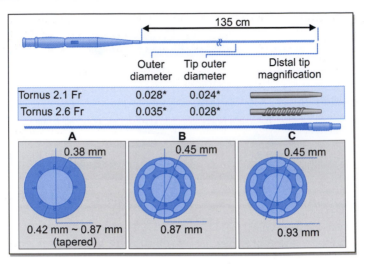

Fig. 12.34: Tornus microcatheter

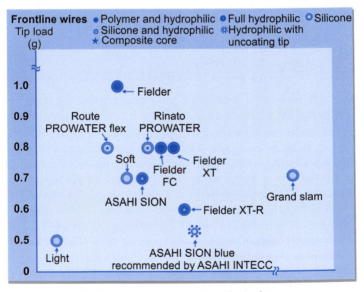

Fig. 12.35: CTO wires: Fielder, Miracle, Confianza

selective applications (e.g. Instent restenosis, calcified lesions, microchannels).

- *Core taper material:* Shorter tapers for improved torque response. Stainless steel increases torque transmission.
- *Core diameter:* Larger for increased support and torque response.
- *Coatings:* Hydrophilic for tracking (body) and hydrophobic for torque response (near tip).

Special CTO Wires

Japanese operators have revolutionized CTO Intervention and we have learned different functions of the wires used in CTO and based on that wires can be classified as shown (Fig. 12.35):

- *Penetrators:* Which can penetrate the proximal cap and seek microchannels and cross the CTOs. They usually have tapered tip, hydrophilic coated spring coil attached to the tip (joint-less) leading to unique torque transmission.
  Fielder FC, XT, Gaia 1
  Conquest Pro (tip load 8-20 g), Gaia 2 (tip load 3.5 g).
- *Sliders:* Hydrophilic either spring coil or polymer sleeve or both, they can seek the microchannels and cross CTO (particularly with nipple present) In-stent restenosis, Calcified lesions, Star technique (less tactile feeling).
  Whisper, Pilot (Abott), PT Series (Boston), Fielder (Asahi), Shinobi (J & J).
- *Drillers:* Wires to be rotated in a 90⁰ arc to and fro to cross, used in most CTOs with discrete entry point, after initial attempt with soft or hydrophilic wires (a workhorse technique) may be used for parallel wire technique.
  Miracle wires (thicker spring coil, thicker core wires, shorter length of spring coil).

Special wires for tortuous and calcified CTOs were developed recently, named Gaia 1 and 2 (Asahi). They have very special features, like–
- Tapered tip—0.010 inch/0.011 inch
- Slip coat coating—400 mm (long)
- Double coil structure at the tip
- Round core design with microcone tip.
  These wires unlike other hydrophilic wires have much better torque control and tip direction.

Summary

- Tapered guidewires (plastic jacketed and soft—FIELDER XT) are currently the first choice for antegrade approach. They basically seek and track the micro-channels and cross CTOs. Being floppy they are not suitable in CTOs without micro-channels or tortuous CTOs. Next important wire is PILOT-50, best suited in tapered proximal cap, partial or completely visible micro-channel. If they cannot pass through a microchannel within 10–15 minutes, the wire should be promptly exchanged.
- If FIELDER-XT fails, PILOT-200 would be the best wire to travel within the occluded segment with support of microcatheter.
- If the target artery is tortuous, either miracle wires (3, 4.5 or 6 g) or Gaia 2 can be selected, Gaia 2 is an excellent wire with 3.5 g tip load and excellent torque transmission and is the wire of choice in passing along tortuous arteries and entering fine channels.
- If the target artery is relatively straight, the tapered floppy guidewire may be exchanged with conquest pro like wires. Limiting the number of wires will help the operator to build up confidence and improve understanding with tactile feedback and behavior of each wire.

Other Techniques

Parallel wire technique (see Fig. 12.36):
1. One moderately stiff wire, if that goes into a false channel.
2. Another stiffer wire taken and tried to negotiate in a different path.

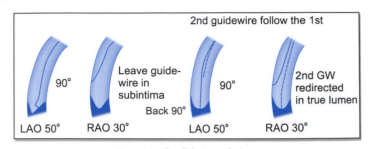

Fig. 12.36: Parallel wire technique

A useful tip for manipulating a guidewire towards and through a CTO is to coordinate rotational movements made with right hand and forward-backward movements made by the left hand. The rotational movement will seldom cross more than 90°. If the guidewire enters the subintimal space, the wire will feel 'trapped' and this can be confirmed by withdrawal of the wire. Entry into the subintimal space should be determined as soon as possible since the situation can probably be corrected withdrawing the wire and attempting rewiring. It is difficult to enter the right track from a false track because every time the wire goes into the false track. Parallel wiring can help in this situation.

When performing parallel wire technique, the operator should keep the first wire into subintimal space and take the second wire; superimpose the two guidewires on each other in a certain view and then obtain another view at angle of 90° to the first view. If this can be achieved, a simple two-dimensional movement will lead the guidewire back into the intimal space (Muramatsu, 2013).

In the parallel wire techniques a support catheter is used only for one guidewire whereas in a variation of parallel wire technique called 'see-saw' technique, two microcatheters (or OTW balloons) are used to support both guidewires. Some rules of parallel wire technique are:
1. Second guidewire should not be 'spinned' for fear of intertwining.
2. Tip of the 2nd wire should be shaped according to the path it should traverse.
3. Early redirection of the wire within CTO is important to create a new pathway.

Side branch technique: If the wire enters the side branch, then balloon dilatation along that path may open the main branch track.

When there is a dissection at the CTO distal cap, the antegrade wire may cross one of the branches, whereas wiring of the other branch may be challenging.

Prolonged antegrade wiring attempts with a second guidewire may cause dissection of the other branch ostium and side branch occlusion. Balloon dilatation (Fig. 12.37A) along the side branch may open the path towards MB or keeping the balloon inflated at the ostium of SB (Fig. 12.37B), 2nd wire may be tried to enter the MB. Hair pin wire (reverse wire) (Fig. 12.37C) technique is also described to direct the tip of the wire to the MB. In this technique a polymer jacketed wire is bent approximately 3 cm from the wire tip and advanced into the SB and then pulled back to enter MB.

Special Situations

IVUS guidance in CTO: The main disadvantage for IVUS guidance of CTO intervention is the lateral view of the IVUS probe. A prototype of

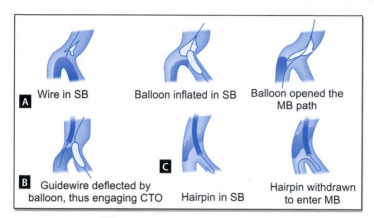

Figs 12.37A to C: Side branch techniques

forward looking IVUS system was developed but till now it has never been commercialized. IVUS can help during wire introduction to the proximal fibrous cap of CTO in presence of SB and from this location the wire reaching the origin of total occlusion can be visualized. IVUS can also help with reintroduction of the wire from false lumen to true lumen, but it is necessary to introduce the IVUS probe to the false lumen after its predilatation with small balloon. This technique unfortunately increases the risk of vessel perforation.

STAR Technique

Retrograde approach: Involves advancement of a guidewire and a micro-catheter through a collateral vessel into the distal true lumen, followed by occluded segment crossing and subsequent antegrade or retrograde wire true lumen placement with various subintimal tracking.

- Identify the donor artery giving collaterals to the distal segment of the artery which is proximally occluded CTO.
- Next is identification of right collaterals. Collaterals may be of two types—septal and epicardial. Besides, bypass grafts are sometimes used for Post-CABG (coronary artery bypass grafting) cases to open CTO retrogradely.
- Of the collaterals, septal collaterals are the best conduits for retrograde approach as they are straight, direct and do not usually cause tamponade, if perforated accidentally. Whereas epicardial collaterals are lengthy, tortuous, fragile and more prone to perforation and development of tamponade.
- *Guide catheter:* Usually, 90 cm guide catheter is necessary (6 F or 7 F). If shorter guide catheter is not available, one can cut the guide catheter to make it shorter (Fig. 12.38)
- *ACT:* An activated clotting time of 300-350 sec. should be targeted, especially when retrograde equipments are in place, to reduce the risk of catheter-induced thrombosis. It should be verified every 20-30 minutes.
- *Collateral access:* Best view is RAO-Cranial, the classic septal collateral connecting LAD and PDA has a classic 'b' shaped distal turn near the connection. These scores should be looked for when advancing the wire. Corsair 150 is the choicest microcatheter (Fig. 12.39).

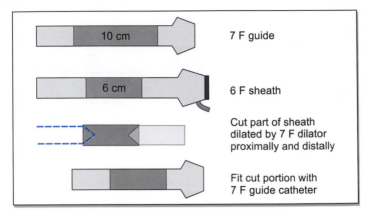

Fig. 12.38: Shortening of guide catheter

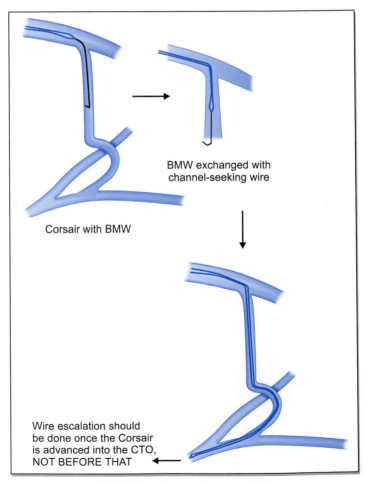

Fig. 12.39: Retrograde wiring using Corsair

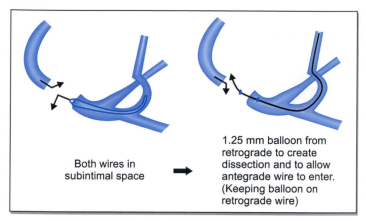

Fig. 12.40: CART technique

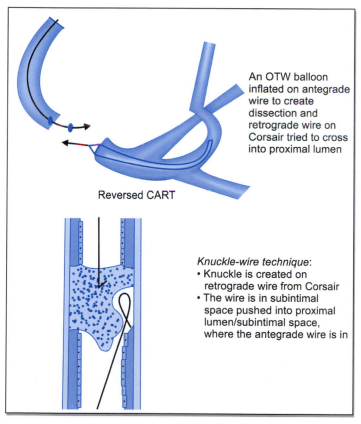

Fig. 12.41: Reversed CART and Knuckle wire

- Crossing CTO (Figs 12.40 and 12.41)
- *Externalization:* In most instances, it is the retrograde wire that crosses into the proximal true lumen. The goal at this point is to orient the retrograde wire into the antegrade guide catheter (Fig. 12.42)

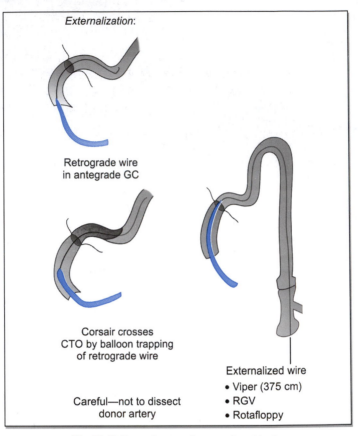

Fig. 12.42: Externalization of retrograde guidewire

- *Opening the occlusion:*
  - Move the Corsair to the distal end of CTO
  - Balloon on the externalized wire into CTO—Predilate (never touch the corsair with distal end of balloon)
  - Workhorse wire through antegrade guide catheter
  - Retrieve the corsair by clockwise and anticlockwise wire rotation alternately, until it reaches the antegrade guide catheter
  - Stent the lesion from antegrade approach.

STAR Technique and Other Dissection-based Approaches

- A consistent message from the literature is that the need of sub-intimal tracking increases with anatomical complexities of CTO. It is found that subintimal tracking is necessary in long calcified CTOs (high J-CTO score), in particularly postcoronary artery bypass grafting patients to get a successful result. Subsequently, the authors have demonstrated, a high rate of repeat revascularization in a small cohort of patients where a subintimal approach occurred.
- Sub-intimal tracking and re-entry (STAR) procedures are associated with poor outcomes because with STAR, re-entry is uncontrolled, unpredictable and run-off is frequently poor, leading to a high likelihood of re-occlusion of target vessel.

- Current dissection based re-entry is different from STAR technique. In contemporary retrograde dissection and re-entry the limit of dissection should be within the confines of CTO lesion. Similarly, controlled antegrade dissection and re-entry limits any dissection plane from within the CTO segment to just beyond the distal cap. The key difference between current procedures and historical STAR techniques is that run-off after successful hybrid CTO-PCI is good and crucially to all distal branches.
- Hybrid CTO operators select cases based on clinical indications and not anatomical features. Once cases have been chosen on clinical need, the hybrid CTO approach is usually algorithm-based strategy, where the CTO anatomy determines the choice of approach which aims for safest, quickest and successful result.

Most Common Reasons for Failure in CTO-PCI

- Use of only one antegrade guide catheter (always have contra-lateral injection)
- Performance of excessive antegrade injection leading to dissections, vessel hematoma and perforation
- Wrong and long curve at the tip of CTO guidewire
- Wrong guidewire selection
- Failure of decision making—when to switch from antegrade to retrograde and vice versa.

Thrombus-containing Lesions

Thrombus is a sensitive, dynamic process which demands accurate classification and compulsive management. Optional angiographic visualization of thrombus is the first step. Thrombus is labile and its grading is better done after crossing the thrombotic lesion with a guidewire. Often there is no change in thrombus grade, but thrombus grade 5 most commonly is down sized after wire passage. Thrombus burden affects clinical outcome. Compared to small thrombus burden (0–1), large thrombus burden (Grade-4) is an important predictor of mortality and MACE.

If the thrombus is small (Grade 0–1), direct angioplasty and stenting may be sufficient. Moderate thrombus burden (Grade 2–3)—warrants pretreatment with an aspiration catheter. Large thrombus burden (Grade 4–5) are challenging. Organized and dense thrombus in late presenting STEMI patient can be extremely difficult cases and their management—from crossing the impenetrable lesions to debulking them, requires considerable skills and often pharmacological help and other devices (Table 12.10 and Figs 12.43 and 12.44).

Table 12.10: Effect of thrombus burden on outcome

	Small thrombus burden (n=567)	Large thrombus burden (n=225)	P-value
Distal emboli	3.5%	17.3%	< 0.001
No reflow	0.5%	4.0%	< 0.001
Final TIMI-III flow	94.9%	83.6%	< 0.001
Myocardial blush grade	53.2%	35.4%	< 0.001

Source: Sianos, JACC, August, 2007

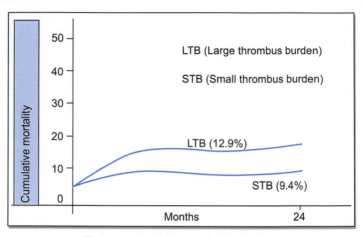

Fig. 12.43: Cumulative mortality in LTB and STB

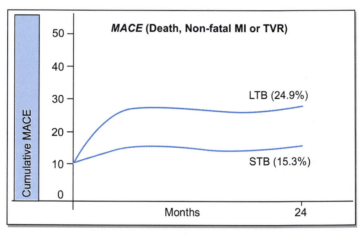

Fig. 12.44: Cumulative MACE in LTB and STB

Large thrombus burden can be anticipated, if:
- Thrombus has greatest linear dimension more than 3 times the RD (reaching distance)
- Cut-off pattern (lesion morphology with an abrupt cut-off without tapering before occlusion)
- Presence of accumulated thrombus (5 mm of linear dimension) proximal to the lesion
- Presence of floating thrombus proximal to the occlusion
- Persistent contrast medium distal to the obstruction
- Reference lumen diameter of the IRA > 4 mm.

Thrombus burden in coronary artery can also affect incidence of stent thrombosis after implantation of drug-eluting stent (Fig. 12.45).

How to tackle moderate to large thrombus burden? Thrombus causing disaster during PCI results from distal migration of the particles clogging the microcirculation by preventing the blood flow reaching the myocardial cells. Theoretically, thrombus can be managed by thrombus busters (thrombectomy), thrombosuction (thrombosuction

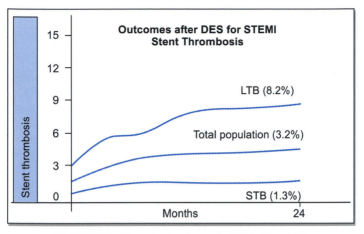

Fig. 12.45: Stent thrombosis outcome for DES in LTB and STB

catheters) and preventing thrombus to migrate distally (protection devices).

Mainly thrombus containing lesions are anticipated in native coronary arteries during acute myocardial infarction and in cases of saphenous vein graft intervention.

Experience about these devices in different clinical situations resulted in selection of them as adjunct (Class-IIa for manual Thrombosuction in Acute Myocardial Infarction and Class-I for distal protection devices in SVG intervention).

Acute Myocardial Infarction

Primary angioplasty and stenting is the principal method of reperfusion in acute ST elevation myocardial infarction.

The procedure is still evolving to have a perfect result. The guidelines getting changed with changing directions due to huge number of information which is piling up every year. The histopathologic hall mark of acute myocardial infarction is plaque rupture and attendant thrombus formation which can be occlusive resulting ST elevation MI. The primary goal would be to remove thrombus before stenting to reduce distal embolization and to improve flow and visualization. Theoretically, this should enhance myocardial perfusion and facilitate procedural success. In observational studies higher thrombus burden is seen to be associated with higher stent thrombosis rate.

Early trials supported this concept and even demonstrated mortality benefit to upfront routine thrombus aspiration in primary PCI (TAPAS Trial 2008). However, later studies (TASTE, 2013 and TOTAL, 2015) have dimmed enthusiasm.

So, in ACC-AHA-SCAI focused update on Primary PCI for patients with ST elevation myocardial infarction placed routine manual thrombosuction before Primary PCI as Class-III (not useful) and they placed it as Class-IIb in bailout situations like initially unplanned but later used during the procedure because of unsatisfactory initial result or procedural complication, analogous to the definition of 'bailout' glycoprotein IIb/IIIa use.

What would be the Place of Manual Thrombosuction?

Many authorities believe following will be the indications for selective use of manual aspiration thrombectomy:

- Large visible thrombus burden (Butman, 2016, CCI)
- Acute myocardial infarction with ectatic IRA with thrombus (Butman, 2016, CCI)
- Late onset ST elevation myocardial infarction (St. Desch, JACC, 2016)
- Bailout situations.

Another issue came up during this focused guideline, especially depending on 4 RCTS (STEMI-17, PRAMI, CULPRIT, DANAMI-3) that is whether significant lesion in non-IRA should be treated during primary PCI in hemodynamically stable patients. In 2011 guidelines it was Class-III, now it has been changed to IIb. The writing committee emphasizes that the change should not be interpreted as endorsing the runtime performance of multivessel PCI in all patients of ST elevation myocardial infarction and multivessel disease.

Actually in hemodynamically stable patients, recommendations in the 2013 STEMI guideline with regard to PCI of a noninfarct artery at a time separate from primary PCI in patients who have spontaneous symptoms and myocardial ischemia or who have intermediate or high risk findings on noninvasive testing remain operative.

Manual Thrombosuction Catheters

Key features of an aspiration catheter are:

1. Deliverability
2. Kink resistance
3. Aspiration power.

Its basic structure is a dual-channel catheter. One channel from the tip is for guidewire, other channel is for aspiration. Initial catheters were less deliverable and were liable to be kinked. Newer catheters are hydrophilic coated, some are with stylets and kink resistant (Fig. 12.46).

The comparative summary of different catheters are given in Table 12.11.

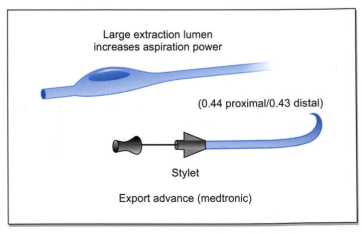

Fig. 12.46: Manual thrombosuction catheter

Table 12.11: The competitive summary of different catheters

Stylet based	Manufacturer	Product
Eliminate	Terumo	
Pronto LP	Vascular solutions	
Thrombuster–III GR	Kareka	
Thrombuster–II	Atrium	
Nonstylet based		
Quick cat	Kensey Nash	
Pronto V3	Vascular solutions	

Almost all catheters are of similar advantages or disadvantages, any one of them can be used. But it is better to get used to any one of them so, that no hiccups are encountered during their use in a very crucial time.

Technique of manual thrombosuction (during primary PCI):
1. If there is TIMI-0 or TIMI-I flow—manual thrombosuction should be performed.
2. Aspiration should be started 2 cm before the lesion.
3. Thrombosuction catheter then should be moved very slowly with continuous aspiration and the lesion should be passed, if possible.
4. Risk of distal embolization increases, if:
   a. Performed too quickly
   b. Retrograde pattern (passing the lesion by thrombectomy catheter and then pulling it back with aspiration).
5. Perform aspiration slowly—use 2nd or 3rd syringe.
6. Two or three passages are recommended.
   A flow chart of thromboaspiration is provided (Flow chart 12.5).

Large Bulky Thrombus

Large bulky thrombus (LBT) responds poorly to thrombus aspiration catheters. In fact in many instances these catheters aspirate only up to 20% of the total thrombus burden. In dealing with LBT, establishing TIMI-III flow should be the primary aim. This will lead to ST resolution and reperfusion. Stenting in such situation could deteriorate the flow due to distal embolization. So, stents may be deferred till the thrombus load is dissolved and situation improves.

What do you do in such cases?
1. Manual thrombo-suction
2. Intracoronary tenecteplase

Flow chart 12.5: Thromboaspiration use

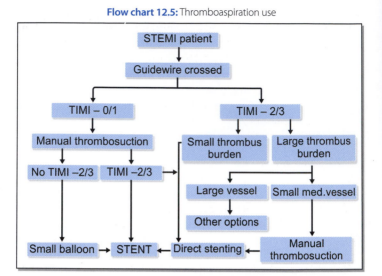

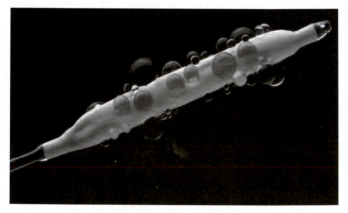

Fig. 12.47: Clearway catheter

- Microporous PTFE balloon mounted on a 2.7 Fr Rx catheter
- Fluid weeps through the pores—no high pressure jets
- Vessel occlusion—site-specific infusion without systemic drug dilution from preferential flow to the LCX or aorta (blowback)

3. *Intracoronary tenecteplase:* In conjunction to mechanical intervention, tenecteplase (TNK) was seen successful in dissolving angiographic thrombus and/or improving flow in 91% of patients (Kelly RV, 2005) (Dose range 5–25 mg).

4. *Intracoronary GP 2b 3a receptor blockers:* Intracoronary abciximab is found to be useful (0.25 mg/kg) in patients with large thrombus burden. Even small molecules (double bolus of eptifibatide 180 μg each or tirofiban 10 μg/kg) have shown benefits. Infusion rather than bolus of abciximab with clearway catheters (Fig. 12.47) showed benefit in recent trials.

5. *Deferred stenting:* During primary PCI an IRA with LBT where thrombosuction and intracoronary drugs are given but still the flow is not optimum, a deferred stent strategy, 4–16 hours after the primary

procedures (DEFER STEMI) can be undertaken safely. Although the concept needs to be evaluated in a randomized setting, it seems both safe and efficacious resulting in a low rate of MACE and high level of myocardial salvage determined by CMR.

6. M-Guard.

Embolic protection devices:

There are four basic classes of EPDs categorized according to their mechanism of operation:

1. Distal occlusion
2. Distal filter
3. Proximal occlusion
4. Local plaque trapping (M-Guard).

US Food and Drug Administration (FDA) approval of the first such device (the distal occlusion guardwire, medtronic, vascular) was predicted on a 42% reduction in 30 days Major Adverse Coronary Event (MACE) rates in a large randomized trial of Saphenous Vein Coronary Artery Bypass Graft PCI, as compared with stenting over a convention guidewire without EPD. This showed consistent benefit independent of GPIIbIIIa receptor antagonist use, across lesion subgroups at varying risk for MACE based on angiographic quantification of graft degeneration and estimated lesion plaque volume. It established EPD as the standard care for SVG Stenting with favorable cost-benefit ratio. One of the limitations of using EPD was that it blocked the flow across the graft sometimes causing ischemia leading to introduction of distal filters. The distal filters for embolic protection depends on the concept that deployed filter can allow ongoing perfusion yet trap some, if not all, particulate debris.

The filters usually have pore size of 100 μm, but they track even smaller particles. Experimental data suggest that embolic particles < 100 μm are tolerated in far larger number before interfering with microcirculatory function than are larger particles. More over the clinical confirmation of equivalency of some distal filters and distal occlusion devices to the guardwire distal occlusion device and ease of use, maintenance of distal perfusion and the possibility of contrast imaging during procedure have made the filter the first choice in SVG stenting (Fig. 12.48).

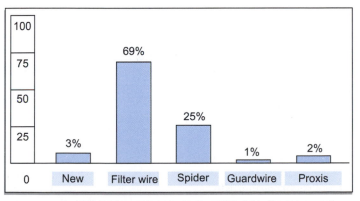

Fig. 12.48: International MD Survey 2009 (Preferred EPD).
(*Source*: Mahmood A., Cath Cardiovasc Int: 2012;79: 834-42)

A Few Words about SVG Angioplasty

Degeneration and occlusion of saphenous vein grafts continue to be significant problems in maintaining long-term benefits in patients who have undergone coronary artery bypass grafting surgery. SVG occlusion during the 1st year is as high as 15%, and 10 years patency is only 60%. SVG failure is associated with a significant increase in MACE including death, myocardial infarction and the need for repeat revascularization.

SVG disease occurs in 3 phases

Early (before hospital discharge), intermediate (1 month–1 year) and late (beyond 1 year).

Early graft failure is due to thrombotic closure usually at the site of anastomosis as a result of endothelial injury and the release of inflammatory cytokines during surgery. Technical factors, such as poor distal run-off, graft kinking and small target vessel diameter, predispose grafts to early occlusion. After the first month, exposure of the vein grafts to arterial pressure results in neointimal hyperplasia. The pathophysiological process causes intimal damage, fibrosis, platelet aggregation, the release of growth factors and smooth muscle cell proliferation. After the first year, aggressive atherosclerotic narrowing occurring over the already abnormal endothelium is the main mechanism for the graft failure.

Atherosclerotic plaques in SVGs are more diffuse, friable and contain more foam and inflammatory cells, have absent or thin fibrous caps and little or no calcification in comparison to native coronary atherosclerosis. These characteristics predispose SVGs to extensive thrombotic burden and distal embolization during intervention.

What should you remember while doing a PCI in SVG? ACC/AHA—2011

- Native grafted vessel PCI is better than PCI in degenerated SVG
- Embolic protection devices should be used in SVG intervention when technically feasible (Class I B)
- PCI is not recommended for chronic SVG occlusions (Class III C)
- GPIIb/IIIa inhibitors are not beneficial as adjunct (Class III B)
- When technically feasible, PCI should be performed in patients with early ischemia (< 30 days) after coronary artery bypass grafting (Class I)
- PCI is reasonable in patients with ischemia that occurs 1–3 years after CABG and who have preserved LV function with discrete lesions in graft conduits—Class IIa
- PCI is reasonable in patients with diseased vein grafts more than 3 years after coronary artery bypass grafting.
- FFR is not very effective due to high specificity and low sensitivity.

Predictors of MACE for SVG PCI:

- Lesion length and stenosis (> 50%)
- Greater SVG degeneration score (Table 12.12)
- Larger plaque volume
- Female sex
- Chronic kidney disease (CKD)
- Major CK-MB release after SVG PCI is a powerful independent predictor of late mortality.

Ongoing studies are enrolling patients (VALETTI-II) to compare PCI versus medical therapy for reduction of MACE in intermediate

Table 12.12: SVG degeneration score

The SVG degeneration score is a measure of the extent of lumen irregularities and ectasia (>20% of the reference normal segment) within SVG that makes up:		
<25% of total SVG length	=	0
26–50% of total SVG length	=	1
51–75% of total SVG length	=	2
>75% of total SVG length	=	3

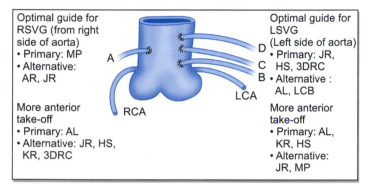

Fig. 12.49: Guide catheter selection in SVG angioplasty
Abbreviations: A, grafts to distal RCA; B, grafts to LAD; C, grafts to diagonals; D, grafts to OM/ramus

lesions (30–60%) in SVG. Though initial small studies show PCI with a drug-eluting stent results in better MACE/TVF in intermediate lesions compared to medical therapy.

Technical Issues

Guide catheter selection: A common selection protocol for choosing guide catheter is based on direction of the graft and size of the aorta. The right-sided grafts are usually lower placed and directed downwards. The left-sided grafts are usually higher placed in the anterior or lateral wall (Fig. 12.49).

Predilatation versus direct stenting: Direct stenting has the potential benefit of trapping debris and decreasing distal embolization that may occur from repeated balloon inflations. A prospective randomized trial is needed to determine whether predilatation VS direct stenting is effective in reducing distal embolization.

Stent sizing: Though there is no prospective randomized study, small stent size (0.9 to 1) is better than smaller and bigger sizes (Fig. 12.50).

Drug-eluting stent versus bare metal stent: Though there is conflicting results in long-term benefit of drug-eluting stent, all these data (Fig. 12.51) underlines the fact that drug-eluting stent can be considered effective and safe at short-term (one year) follow-up as consistently shown in several studies; however, longer term follow-up of adequately performed studies is required to confirm that drug-eluting stent remain safe and effective also after one year (Table 12.13).

These data were formed by combination and meta-analysis of 4 different RCTs, namely, RRISC (75), BASKET (47), (80), ISARCABG (610)

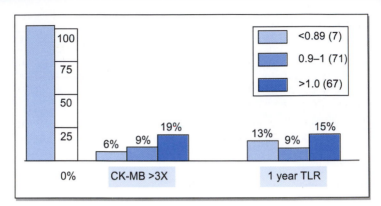

Fig. 12.50: Stent diameter/reference lumen diameter (IVUS)
(*Source:* Hong YJ. Am J Cardiol. 2010;105:179-85.)

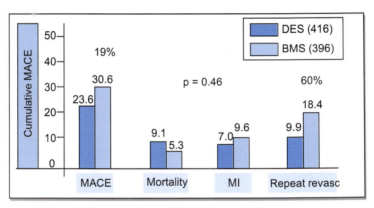

Fig. 12.51: DES vs BMS in SVGs 3 years. Events
(Alam M. Clinic Cardiol. 2012; 35:291-6.)

Table 12.13: Difference between BMS and DES-ISR

Type	Bare metal stent (BMS)-ISR	Drug-eluting stent (DES)-ISR
	Usually diffuse	Usually focal, mostly at the stent edge
Timing	Early (6–8 months)	Delayed (ongoing late loss out to 5 years)
Histopathology		
Smooth muscle cellularity	Rich	Hypocellular
Proteoglycan content	Moderate	High
Peristent fibrin and inflammation	Occasional	Frequent
Complete endothelialization	3–6 months	Up to 48 months
Neoatherosclerosis	Infrequent, late	Relatively frequent accelerated course
Optical coherence tomography	Homogeneous, high signal based	Heterogeneous, layered

In-stent Restenosis

Treatment of in-stent restenosis (ISR) remains a challenge. With increasing number of drug-eluting stent use, the restenosis has come down significantly, but with the phenomenal increase in PCI numbers, interventional cardiologists still do come across many ISR patients in everyday practice.

Definition: Mainly angiographic, namely recurrent diameter stenosis >50% at the stent segment or its edges (5 mm segment proximal and distal to the stent)

Classification (Fig. 12.52)

Pattern – 1	Focal	19%
Pattern – 2	Diffuse	35%
Pattern – 3	Proliferative	50%
Pattern – 4	Occlusion	98%

Though thought as mostly benign, a DES in-stent restenosis particularly may present with unstable symptoms and may precipitate an acute coronary syndrome (ACS). Currently, the functional significance of ISR may be readily evaluated by using fractional flow reserve (FFR). Notably the clinical outcome of patients with in-stent restenosis with deferred interventions based on FFR > 0.75 is excellent.

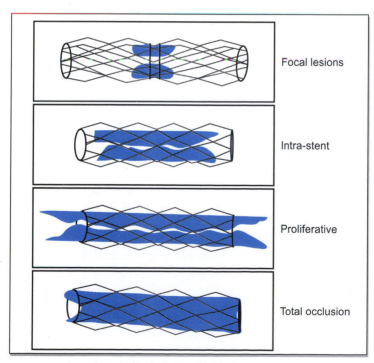

Fig. 12.52: Classification of ISR

Underlying Factors

- Mostly underlying mechanical problems, which is preventable.
- Under expansion (Undersizing/under-deployment)
- Geographical miss (missing plaques)
- Stent fracture (more frequent in right coronary artery)
- Drug resistance and local hypersensitivity.

Role of Intravascular Imaging

Intravascular imaging provides unique insights into the underlying etiology of in-stent restenosis, but its role of optimizing the clinical results of these reinterventions still remained unsettled. But it is generally accepted that one form of intravascular imaging makes the job easier during treatment of in-stent restenosis by PCI.

Balloon Angioplasty

It is one of the earliest strategies used in patients presenting with in-stent restenosis. It may be helpful in some cases of focal in-stent restenosis but restenosis rate is high.

- Balloon: Artery should be 1.1:1
- High pressure dilatation in case of under-expansion
- Balloon slippage (water-melon seeding) is quite disturbing (more in diffuse ISR)
- Mostly used as a predilatation procedure before implantation of another DES or DCB (drug-coated balloon)

Cutting Balloon/Scoring Balloon

- Initial observation studies showed better results than balloon only
- Avoids 'Watermelon seeding' effect
- Scoring balloons are better than cutting balloon in trackability due to their superior flexibility
- Use of these devices before DCB or DES implantation is particularly attractive.

Rotational Atherectomy

Largely replaced by scoring balloons but may still be required as a bailout strategy in patients with undilatable in-stent restenosis as a result of severely under expanded stents or calcified intra-stent neoatherosclerosis.

Repeat Stenting with Drug-eluting Stents (DES)

- DES in case of BMS-ISR is proved to be very effective. Treatment of DES-ISR is challenging and is associated with poorer late outcomes. Acute results are encouraging and even in a focal pattern of DES-ISR, re-treatment with another drug-eluting stent is better than balloon angioplasty, particularly in patients with stent fracture or restenosis extending outside stent edge.
- Drug-switching was initially thought attractive but clinical trials do not support any superiority of switching. Sirolimus DES in-stent restenosis may be treated with any limus, even sirolimus again.

- Second generation drug-eluting stents are better than first generation drug-eluting stents for treatment of DES-in-stent restenosis.
- Bioresorbable scaffolds have also been proposed as treatment of DES-in-stent restenosis. The chief advantage is that device should eventually disappear from the vessel wall avoiding multiple stent layers (onion-skin phenomenon), but the device is bulky, not fit for smaller vessels as well as its radial strength and recoil may be a question.

Drug-coated Balloons

Drug-coated balloons may be a very good treatment options in patients with in-stent restenosis and multiple metal layers, in those with large side branches, and in those at high bleeding risk undergoing prolonged DAPT.

Suggested Reading

1. Agostoni P, Voskuil M. Tools and Techniques: Percutaneous Intervention of Saphenous Vein Graft lesions. Euro Intervention 2013.
2. Carrie D, Oldroyd KG, McEntegart M. A randomized trial of deferred stenting versus immediate stenting to prevent No or slow reflow in Acute STEMI (DEFER-STEMI): JACC. 2014;63(20):2088-95.
3. Current Overview of Rotational Atherectomy: Does Rotablator make sense? www.Emodinamica.gise.it /22/2202.
4. Gallagher S, Ajay K, Jain RA. Archbold Intra-coronary Thrombolytic Therapy: A treatment option for failed mechanical thrombectomy: Catheter Cardiovascular Intervention. 2012;80:835-7.
5. Jayal D, Thompson CA. The Retrograde technique for Recanalization of Chronic Total Occlusions: A Step-by-step approach: JACC. Cardiovascular Interventions. 2012;5(1):1-11.
6. Tak WK, James D, Liow M. Perfection of Precise ostial stent placement. Journal of Invasive Cardiology. 2012;24(7):354-78.

Structural Heart Disease
(Balloon Valvuloplasty)

- Shuvanan Ray

Mitral Balloon Valvuloplasty

Patients with mild to moderate mitral stenosis (MS) who are asymptomatic, frequently remain so for years and clinical outcomes are similar to age matched normal patients. However, symptomatic or severe MS is associated with poor long-term outcomes. If stenosis is not relieved mechanically, intervention should be performed in patients with clinically significant MS (valve area < 1.5 cm²) (Fig. 13.1).

Until the first publication by Inoue and co-workers describing percutaneous mitral commissurotomy in 1984, surgery was the only treatment for patients with mitral stenosis. Since then, a considerable evolution of technique has occurred, and a large number of patients with a wide range of clinical conditions have now been treated.

Selection of patients: Besides symptomatic status, transthoracic echocardiography is the most important investigation for the choice of treatment strategy. Echocardiography plays a central role in the diagnosis and management of MS. Several 2D scoring systems have been suggested for evaluation of mitral valve anatomy. However, none

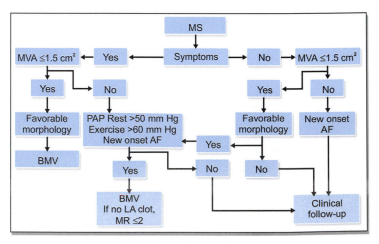

Fig. 13.1: Indication of BMV
Abbreviations: MS, mitral stenosis; MVA, mitral valve area; BMV, balloon mital volvotomy; PAP, pulmonary artery pressure; AF, atrial fibrillation; LA left atrial; MR, mitral regurgitation
(*Source:* Braunwald Heart Disease : 9th Edition—Page 1496)

Table 13.1: Wilkins score

Score	Leaflet mobility	Valve thickness	Subvalvular thickening	Valvular calcification
1.	Highly mobile with little restriction	Normal thickness (4–5 mm)	Minimal chordal thickening	A single area of calcification
2.	Decreases mobility in midportion and base of leaflets	Midleaflet/ marginal thickening	Chordal thickening 1/3 up chordal length	Confined to leaflet margins
3.	Forward movement of valve leaflets in diastole	Total leaflet thickening (5–8 mm)	Chordal thickening 2/3 up chordal lenth	Up to mid-leaflet
4.	No or minimal forward movement of leaflets in diastole	Severe thickening (≥ 8 mm)	Complete chordal thickening to papillary muscle	Throughout most of the valve leaflets

of the available score are shown to be superior to any of the others. Most cardiologists use Wilkins score (Table 13.1), but it has many limitations:

- Assessment of commissural involvement is not included or underestimated
- Does not account for uneven distribution of pathologic abnormalities
- Does not account for relative contribution of each variable (no weightage of variables)
- Frequent underestimation of subvalvular disease.

Status of commissures is also a very important factor determining the prognosis after balloon mitral valvotomy (BMV). The short-axis view of mitral valve can assess the status of the commissures in most of the cases. If there is translucency of both the commissures in short-axis view, it predicts excellent results with well split commissures.

Transesophageal echocardiography (TEE) is also essential for determination of left atrial (LA) clot, if any, and also to study the commissural pattern. Incorporation of 3D in TEE allows interrogation of commissures more directly which is helpful to understand asymmetric fusion or calcification of commissures. Asymmetric deformation of mitral orifice increases the risk of MR with balloon valvuloplasty. The commissural morphology can be assessed and classified according to a score (Sutaria, Heart. 2006:92,52-57; Nobyoshi Circulation. 2009;119:e211-e219):

0 Neither commissure fused or calcification of both commissures or absent fusion of one commissure and calcification of other.

1 Partial fusion of one commissure and absent fusion or calcification of other.

2 Extensive fusion of one commissure and absent fusion or calcification of the other OR partial fusion of both commissures.

3 Extensive fusion of commissures, partial fusion of the other and no commissural calcification.

4 Extensive fusion of both commissures and no commissural calcification.

Higher scores provided a more predictable result. Increase in mitral valve area (MVA) post-BMV was more in patients with higher commissural score (score 3–4). Commissural calcification is a very important factor to determine inefficiency and complication with balloon valvotomy (severe MR).

Contraindications to BMV

- Persistent LA or LA appendage thrombus
- ≥ Grade 2 mitral regurgitation (MR)
- Massive bicommissural calcification
- Severe concomitant aortic valve disease
- Severe organic tricuspid stenosis or severe functional regurgitation with enlarged annulus
- Severe concomitant coronary artery disease, requiring coronary artery bypass grafting.

The Inoue Balloon Catheter

The Inoue device differs substantially from conventional balloons. It is a tri-layered balloon, a nylon mesh is sandwiched between two latex layers to construct the balloon material. The latex layer is extremely compliant, whereas the nylon mesh limits the maximum inflated diameter of the balloon and also gives it its unique shape and inflation characteristics (Figs 13.2A to C).

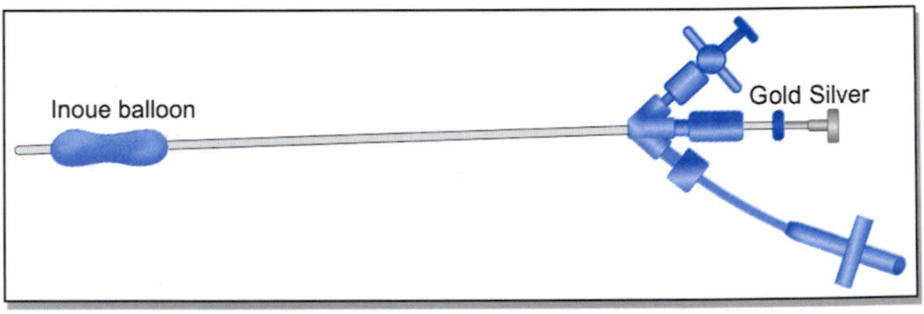

![Inoue balloon catheter with Inoue balloon, Gold Silver markings]

Fig. 13.2A: Inoue balloon catheter

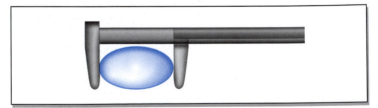

Fig. 13.2B: Caliper

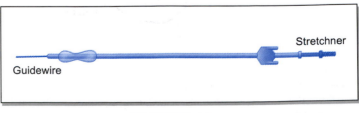

Fig. 13.2C: Stretchner

The intraballoon pressure rises from a "low pressure zone" to "high pressure zone" as the balloon is inflated, within 2 mm of its nominal size, e.g. the 24–26 mm zone in 26 mm balloon catheter. In low pressure zone, the balloon provides 1–2 atm lateral pressure and in high pressure zone, the balloon imparts 2–4 atm pressure. A 26 mm inflation with a 30 mm balloon imparts less lateral pressure than 26 mm inflation with a 26 mm balloon. The balloon can be safely inflated to a maximum diameter of 1 mm above nominal size because of the built-in safety margin. The initial inflation is never to be performed in high pressure zone, rather the inflation should be stepwise.

Sizing of the Balloon

Balloon catheter is selected according to height of the patient in centimeter rounded to nearest zero and dividing it by ten and adding ten to that [e.g. height = 147 cm; then RS = 150 × (1/10) +10 = 25 mm].

Valvular status	Balloon catheter	
Pliable	RS matched (PTMC = 26 for RS = 25 mm)	
Calcified/SL	one size < RS matched (PTMC = 24 for RS = 25 mm)	
Valvular status	Initial	Increments
Pliable	(RS-2) mm	1 mm or 0.5 mm in high pressure zone (if MR or unilateral)
Calcified/SL	(RS-4) mm	1 mm in low pressure zone 0.5 mm in high pressure zone

Balloon Preparation

The balloon catheter comes packaged with all components necessary for the dilatation procedure. This includes a rigid 14F plastic dilator, 0.025 inch spring tip exchange guidewire, a balloon stretching tube, caliper for measuring the balloon diameter, a calibrated inflation series for the balloon and a stylet for manipulating the balloon across the mitral valve after it has been placed in the left atrium. The balloon catheter lumen is flushed with saline. Dilute contrast (4:1) is injected through the vent lumen to purge air from the inflate/deflate channel to the balloon. The precalibrated balloon inflation syringe is filled to calibration corresponding to the smallest inflated diameter and measured with the caliper. If there is mismatch the difference should be noted and adjusted during the second stage of testing, when the balloon is inflated to its nominal diameter. The syringe is then made air free and filled to the calibration corresponding to maximal nominal inflated size. The balloon is inflated and tested to ensure that the maximal size calibration is also proper.

The next step in balloon preparation is to stretch the balloon catheter along its long-axis, causing it to become more slender. The balloon stretcher is inserted into the center lumen of the balloon over the guidewire and advanced until it locks into the metal hub at the proximal end of the balloon (the silver). The silver and stretching tube is advanced into the balloon catheter up to the gold marker. This leaves the balloon in its elongated slenderized form. The guidewire is then removed.

Method 1: Trans-septal Puncture

The most important step of Inoue balloon mitral valvuloplasty is the septal puncture. The puncture should be made at the right spot (fossa ovalis) and the remaining part of the procedure becomes very simple.

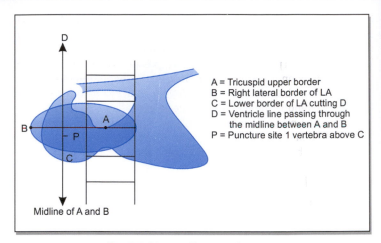

Fig. 13.3: RA angio: Trans-septal puncture

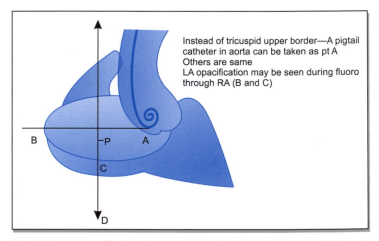

Fig. 13.4: Hung's modification of Inoue's method of trans-septal puncture: No RA angio

And the puncture in an inappropriate atrial septal site may produce cardiac perforation and tamponade or may make the procedure difficult and often unsuccessful.

Inoue derived a method for trans-septal puncture by performing right atrial (RA) angiography in anteroposterior (AP) view and following that up to opacification of LA in levo phase (Fig. 13.3).

Hung et al. modified the Inoue method of RA angiography by putting a pigtail in aortic valve and adjusting the puncture site according to that (Fig. 13.4).

In the lateral projection, locating an appropriate puncture site is less precise as the landmarks in this view depend very much on the left and right atrial sizes. However, the lateral view serves to confirm the appropriate posterior direction of the needle-catheter assembly (Fig. 13.5).

Using anteroposterior and lateral view to puncture, sometimes cannot guarantee against inadvertent puncture of RA or aorta. Right anterior oblique (RAO) 45° view was introduced by AJ Doorey (1991),

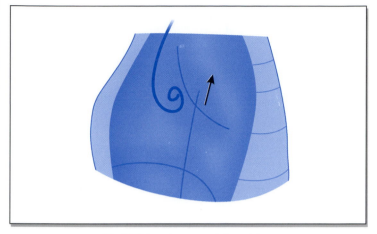

Fig. 13.5: Septal puncture in lateral view

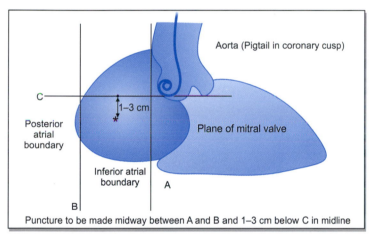

Fig. 13.6: Puncture in RAO view

which gives a more 'enface' view of the septum than the AP view, and puncture minimizes the chance of hitting the posterior atrial wall or aorta (Fig. 13.6).

Steps of Septal Puncture

1. Femoral venous and arterial access on the right side. Sometimes when right femoral venous access is not possible, left femoral vein can be accessed, but it is slightly difficult to orient the septal puncture assembly from the left side
   - Put an 8 F venous sheath and 6 F arterial sheath
   - Do not use heparin till trans-septal puncture is done and LA guidewire is put inside the LA
   - Put a pigtail catheter in the noncoronary cusp of aorta, and put a Terumo guidewire (0.32) in the left brachiocephalic vein. Take a 7 F Mullins sheath/dilator on the wire to the left brachio-cephalic vein

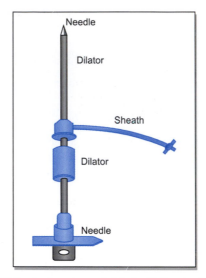

Fig. 13.7: Brockenbrough needle into the Mullins sheath/dilator

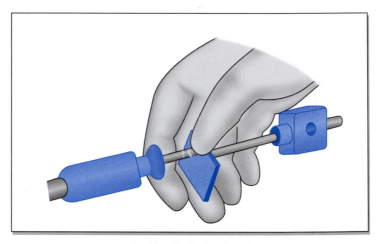

Fig. 13.8: Holding the Brockenbrough needle

- Take a Brockenbrough needle with a 5 cc syringe of contrast attached to the hub into the Mullins sheath/dilator till a few (2–3 mm) of its tip (Fig. 13.7)
- Put a finger (the left index) on the needle between the direction indicator and the catheter hub, to be used as a stopper. This is to prevent the needle from moving forwards and protruding from catheter tip (Fig. 13.8).
- Under frontal fluoroscopic view, the needle-fitted trans-septal catheter with its direction indicator pointing about 4 o'clock is slowly withdrawn downwards till a sudden sharp movement towards the left may be observed, when the tip of the assembly enters fossa ovalis crossing the limbic ledge.
- Now the needle is rotated clockwise with the assembly, so that the direction indicator comes between 4 o'clock and 7 o'clock position and the needle tip rotates at the assumed puncture site.

- Remove left index finger from the needle and push the needle gently—it enters LA and check with contrast.

Few Areas of Trouble

1. The rotation of catheter needle assembly varies with LA size, it is 4 o'clock when LA is small (<4 cm) and 6 o'clock when LA is large (>5 cm), and about 7 o'clock when LA is aneurysmal (>7 cm).
   - In large LA, sometimes the atrial septum bulges towards RA and it is very difficult to align the assembly to midline. In these cases, when tried to rotate from 4 o'clock position, the assembly suddenly moves to 9 o'clock position and the tip moves to right. Tips are:
     - Come a little lower and try to rotate and keep the assembly in the midline
     - Come further out of the catheter with the needle and then rotate the needle clockwise, while rotating the catheter anti-clockwise, with the left hand, pushing it gently to the septum at the puncture site—feel the septal bounce and pierce
     - Make the needle a little curved at the tip, and then repeat the whole procedure
     - If at all, it is not possible to align the assembly at the midline, try as close as possible to the midline. The dictum is not to puncture at a site medial to 'midline' and always avoid too low a puncture. Too low a puncture will involve RA and the LA (stitching phenomenon)
     - If the LA lower border is seen, always puncture above it. If it is not seen, puncture at least 1½ vertebral width above the lower atrial border which is seen, that will avoid stitching phenomenon (leading to massive pericardial tamponade)
   - Inadvertent puncture of aorta, as evident by contrast injection or pressure recording is usually uneventful if the needle is withdrawn immediately. If the catheter is inadvertently advanced in aorta—the patient should be sent to emergency surgery without pulling out the catheter.
   - If the initial effort of puncture is unsuccessful, the needle should be removed from the catheter and the second attempt is begun by repositioning the catheter in the SVC over the guidewire.
2. *Putting the catheter (IBC) into LA:*
   - After atrial septal puncture and placement of the coiled tip guidewire in the LA, the atrial septum as well as the groin is dilated with the 14 F dilator. The wire should be fixed by the assistant while the 14 F dilator should go in 2–3 times to dilate the venous access as well as the atrial septum. Now the Inoue balloon catheter (IBC) is pushed on the guidewire (vertical to the skin) to cross first the groin, then the septum (Fig. 13.9).
   - At this stage, IV heparin 3000 units given.
   - Once the catheter enters the LA, first the gold connector should be released and pulled. The tip of the balloon will then begin to track around the coiled spring guidewire. The balloon stretching tube and spring guidewire are taken out at the catheter, cleaned and prepared for the latter use to aid in balloon removal.

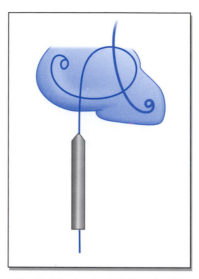

Fig. 13.9: Putting the 14 F dilator into LA

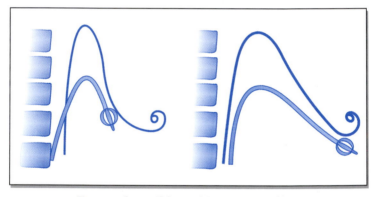

Fig. 13.10: Putting IBC across MV—conventional loop

The balloon catheter can then be flushed and connected to the pressure transducer. The transmitral pressure gradient now can be measured through the balloon catheter and the pigtail catheter pushed into the LV.

3. *Crossing mitral valve by IBC:*
   - The X-ray projection is changed to 30° RAO. The IBC is flushed and LV stylet is introduced to the tip. The distal portion of the IBC is inflated. The stylet is rotated anticlockwise while the IBC is advanced or withdrawn until a bobbing motion is observed. This wood-pecking sign is observed as the balloon moves away from the mitral orifice in systole and towards it in diastole along the axis between mitral orifice and the left ventricular apex. Once the wood-pecking sign is evident, the operator should jerk the LV stylet out during diastole and the IBC crosses the mitral valve.
   - Crossing the mitral valve, the IBC should be negotiated to the LV apex, parallel to the pigtail catheter (Fig. 13.10).

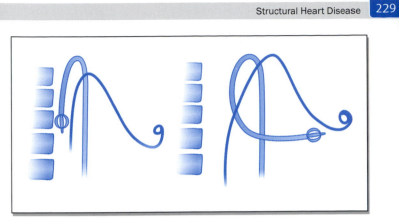

Fig. 13.11: Putting IBC across MV—reverse loop

- The distal part of IBC is now fully dilated and pulled towards MV where it rides over the stenosed valve and then the rest of the IBC is fully dilated and released, which splits the mitral commissures and the valve is dilated.

Alternate Loop Method

If the septal puncture is made medial or cephalic, it is very difficult to align IBC to MV axis, there this loop method works (Fig. 13.11).

Accordion Maneuver

One of the most dreaded complications of BMV is the development of severe MR requiring surgery. Once the MV has been crossed, the free movements of the partially inflated distal balloon in the LV should be ascertained to prevent rupture of chordae, papillary muscles or leaflets, stemming from its subsequent full inflation between chordae. This could happen in presence of severe subvalvular disease which was missed in echocardiography (there a little impression of distal balloon shows deformity of the balloon). In such situations, following things are to be done:

1. By simultaneously pushing the catheter and pulling the stylet in opposite direction (accordion maneuver) to ensure the partially inflated distal balloon slides freely along the orifice-apex axis.
2. In serious subvalvular disease after proper accordion maneuver still there remains a probability of severe MR. There with further dilatation of distal balloon, if it shows deformity (balloon compression sign) then stepwise dilatation should be done. IBC first should be dilated with a smaller size (at least 4 mm less)—presence of MR and commissural split should be assessed, then one should proceed for optimal dilatation (Fig. 13.12).

Postprocedure Evaluation and Balloon Withdrawal

- A favorable result is evident by
  - Reduction of mean transmitral gradient from >10 mm Hg to <5 mm Hg
  - Absence of severe MR.

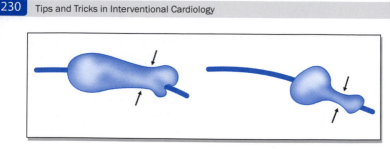

Fig. 13.12: Balloon compression sign

Following dilatation, a left ventriculogram is repeated to finally evaluate MR. The balloon catheter must then be withdrawn across the atrial septum. This is accomplished by re-introducing the balloon stretching tube preloaded with the 0.025 spring-tipped guidewire. The guidewire is advanced and curled in the LA. The balloon stretching tube then locked to the silver connector of the balloon and advanced to the gold connector of the balloon. The IBC becomes straight and is pulled out with the wire.

Pulmonary Balloon Valvuloplasty

Congenital pulmonary valve stenosis comprises of 7.5–9% of all congenital heart disease. Pulmonary valve stenosis may vary from a 'dome' shaped valve during systole to pulmonary ring hypoplasia and dysplastic pulmonary valve. Pulmonary balloon valvuloplasty is now the first option in the management of pulmonary valve stenosis.

Indications

- Moderate to severe of pulmonary valve stenosis (peak-to-peak gradient >50 mm Hg) with normal cardiac index.
- Asymptomatic people with such gradient should be included as indication, if:
  - Poor response to exercise
  - Potential to develop myocardial fibrosis.
- Dysplastic valves are not the ideal candidates, but still can be tried with balloon 1.4–1.5 times the annular size (the determinant of success is the presence of commissural fusion).
- *Selection of balloon catheter*: Many balloons evolved for the purpose from the initial period. Recently, most of the operators use Tyshak-II balloon catheters because of their low profile and excellent trackability. Other balloon catheters which are used are as follows:
  - Tyshak X, Z Med X and II X (Numed, Hopkinton, NY)
  - Inoue balloon catheter (Toray, Japan).
- *Balloon diameter*: Initial recommendations were to use balloons that are 1.2–1.4 times the pulmonary valve annulus. Balloons >1.5 times should not be used for the fear of RV outflow damage.
- In most of the cases, balloons 1.2–1.25 times the pulmonary annulus should be used because they provide good relief of pulmonary valve obstruction while at the same time prevent significant pulmonary regurgitation.

- *Balloon length*: Generally in neonates and infants 20 mm, in children 30 mm and in adults 40 mm long balloon are used. Shorter balloons may pop-out of valve during inflation.
- *Single versus double balloon*: When the pulmonary valve annulus is too large to dilate with a single balloon, two balloons are used across the pulmonary valve for simultaneous inflation. Effective balloon diameter will be 0.8 (D1 + D2) [D1 and D2 are diameters of the balloons used].
- *Technique*: The diagnosis and assessment of pulmonary valve stenosis are made by clinical, radiographic, ECG and Echo-Doppler data. Once a moderate to severe obstruction is diagnosed, cardiac catheterization and cineangiography are performed to consider balloon dilatation of valve.
- *Sedation*: In infants, below 3 months, general anesthesia with endotracheal intubation is used. In children, many operators use ketamine/intermittent doses of midazolam/or fentanyl.
- *Vascular access*: Femoral veins are used mostly but in absence of femoral route transjugular/axillary can be used safely. An arterial line should be maintained for continuous BP monitoring.
- *Hemodynamic assessment and cineangiography*:
  - Swan-Ganz catheter is used to assess all the right-sided pressures from PCW to RA, to calculate peak to peak gradient across pulmonary valve. Simultaneous recording of the RV and femoral artery pressure is also undertaken. RV peak systolic pressure >75% of peak systolic systemic pressure is considered significant for valve dilatation.
  - Biplane/lateral view of the right ventricular outflow tract (RVOT) is performed to assess the annular size and the position of the annulus is marked in respect to any bony point (e.g. sternum and vertebra).
  - Usually, the pulmonary valve is crossed by a Swan ganz catheter (sometimes Cobra, 4 F JR) and a guidewire is placed across the valve. In neonates and young infants, an extra support 0.014 coronary floppy tipped guidewire is placed preferably through the ductus into the descending aorta.
  - In children and adults, an Amplatz SuperStiff guidewire (exchange length) is used to park in distal left or right pulmonary artery.
  - The selected balloon angioplasty catheter is advanced over the guidewire, but within the sheath and positioned across the pulmonary valve using the fixed bony landmarks. For double balloons, femoral veins of both sides are used, two guidewires and then balloons are placed across the pulmonary valve. The balloon is inflated with diluted contrast medium (1 in 4) by an indeflator. The pressure is elevated up to manufacturer-recommended pressure or until disappearance of waist.
- Inoue balloon catheter (IBC) is usually used in adult patient in large annulus were a single balloon inflation can relieve obstruction. The balloon has a dumbbell-like character where it can ride the annulus/obstruction perfectly and can be inflated.
  - The IBC is selected with its maximum diameter not exceeding annular diameter.

- The pulmonary valve is crossed with Swan ganz catheter and a 270 cm 0.025 floppy tipped stainless steel guidewire is placed in pulmonary artery from right femoral vein.
- The groin is dilated with Inoue dilator and the IBC with metal stretcher is placed in RA and the metal tube is removed and the balloon becomes flexible to cross pulmonary valve. The distal end of the balloon sometimes inflated a little to allow the balloon to float across the valve. The balloon is inflated first to a diameter of 3–4 mm < maximal diameter. If the gradient is not successfully reduced it can be inflated up to its maximal diameter.

- *Postprocedure*: After balloon dilatation following parameters are measured:
  - Gradient across pulmonary valve
  - Oxygen saturation
  - Simultaneous RV and femoral artery pressure
    » If the gradient >30 mm Hg—repeat dilatation with a larger balloon (+ 2 mm)
    » After the procedure, a cineangiography is done to assess mobility of the pulmonary valve leaflets, to visualize the jet of constant flow across dilated pulmonary valve, to detect infundibular stenosis and pulmonary regurgitation.

Suggested Reading

1. Cavalcarte JL, Rodriguez L. Role of echocardiography in percutaneous mitral valve intervention. JACC Cardiovascular Imaging. 2012;5(7):733-46.
2. Doorey AJ, Goldenberg EM. Trans-septal catheterization in adults: Enhanced efficiency and safety by low volume operators using a 'Non-standard' technique: Catheterization and Cardiovascular Diagnosis. 1991;22:239:43.
3. Feldman T, Inoue K. Percutaneous Trans-venous Mitral Commissurotomy using Inoue Balloon Catheter. Catheterization and Cardiovascular Diagnosis. 1993;28:119-25.
4. Hung JS. Atrial septal puncture technique in percutaneous trans-venous mitral commissurotomy: Mitral Valvuloplasty using Inoue balloon catheter technique. Catheterization and Cardiovascular Diagnosis. 1992;26:275-84.
5. Kisslo J. NHLBI Balloon Valvuloplasty Registry: Doppler echo evaluation of mitral stenosis pre and post Valvuloplasty (Abstr). J Am Coll Cardiol. 1989;13:114A.
6. Lau KW, Hung JS. Pulmonary valvuloplasty in adults using Inoue balloon catheter: catheterization and cardiovascular diagnosis. 1993;29:99-104.
7. Lin SC, Hwang JJ, Hsu KL. Balloon Pulmonary Valvuloplasty in Adults with Congenital Valvular Pulmonary stenosis. Acta Cardiol Sin: 2004;20:147-53.
8. Oh JK, Seward J.B, Tajik AJ. The Echo Manual, 3rd Edition. Mayo Foundation, 2006.
9. Rao PSS. Percutaneous Balloon Pulmonary Valvuloplasty: State-of-Art. Catheterization and Cardiovascular Intervention. 2007;69:743-64.

Congenital Heart Disease
(Intervention in Adults: ASD/VSD/PDA)

■ Sanjeev S Mukherjee

Device Closure

This chapter is aimed at practically approaching percutaneous closure of cardiac shunts. Reader is advised to refer to textbooks for understanding pathology and further details.

Atrial Septal Defect Closure

Introduction

The most common types of defects in the atrial septum are ostium secundum, ostium primum, sinus venosus and patent foramen ovale. Ostium primum and sinus venosus defects require surgical intervention because of associated defects (cleft in mitral valve causing mitral regurgitation in the ostium primum defects and partial anomalous pulmonary venous connection in sinus venosus defects). The indications to intervene on patent foramen ovale are debated. Some early studies were interpreted to show no major benefit, if surgical closure was performed in adulthood. Based on more recent analysis, it would appear that ASDs should be closed when indicated even in adult and elderly subjects.

Data to Support ASD Closure in Adults

Konstantinides et al. did a 10 years follow-up study in patients with atrial septal defects who underwent surgical closure or medical management. They had 179 patients who were well matched into 2 groups. The 10 years survival rate was 95% in the surgery group and 84% in the non-surgery group. Surgery also appears to have prevented deterioration of the patients' in NYHA functional class.

Salehian et al. evaluated cardiac function following ASD closure. They had 25 patients at a mean age of 46 years, who were studied prior to and 3 months (mean) after device closure. Their right ventricular myocardial performance index (MPI) improved. The lack of improvement of the right ventricular MPI following surgical closure is attributed to the adverse effects of cardiopulmonary bypass on ventricular function.

Brochu et al. showed improvement in VO$_2$ maximum in 37 patients (mean age 49 years), six months after ASD closure, suggesting improvement in functional capacity.

Murphy et al. after studying 123 patient concluded that earlier the closure, better is the 27 years survival rates, emphasizing early intervention in hemodynamically insignificant ASD.

What to do—Device or Surgery?

Although surgical closure of ASDs is safe and effective with low mortality, the morbidity associated with sternotomy/thoracotomy is unavoidable. Most studies comparing surgical versus device closures suggest similar effectiveness, but device closure is less invasive, required no cardio-pulmonary bypass, has less complications (10% vs 31%), requires shorter hospital stays in properly selected patient subgroups. Thus, device closure is now an established practice in most cardiac centers worldwide. I would suggest using only amplatzer septal occluder in the initial few cases due to safety records and ease of manipulation.

Indications

American Heart Association guidelines for closure of ASD

Class-I

1. Transcatheter secundum ASD closure is indicated in patients with hemodynamically significant ASD with suitable anatomic features (Level of evidence: B).

Class-IIa

1. It is reasonable to perform transcatheter secundum ASD closure in patients with transient right to left shunting at the atrial level who have experienced sequelae of paradoxical emboli such as stroke or recurrent transient ischemic attack (Level of evidence: B).
2. It is reasonable to perform transcatheter secundum ASD closure in patients with transient right to left shunting at the atrial level who are symptomatic because of cyanosis and who do not require such a communication to maintain adequate cardiac output (Level of evidence: B).

Class-IIb

1. Transcatheter closure may be considered in patients with a small secundum ASD who are believed to be at risk of thromboembolic events (e.g. patients with a transvenous paring system or chronic indwelling intravenous catheters, patients with hypercoagulable status) (Level of evidence: B).

Contraindications

1. Pulmonary vascular resistance (PVR) in excess of 7 wood units.
2. Acute or recent sepsis or contraindications for antiplatelets therapy.

Evaluation of Defect

Factors that decide suitability for transcatheter closure include size of defect and presence of adequate tissue rims around the defect. Accurate imaging is accomplished using two-dimensional (2D) and three-dimesional (3D) echocardiography and of late, intracardiac echocardiography (ICE). We would focus on comprehensive imaging through transesophageal echocardiography (TEE) for transcatheter closure of ASD.

Definition of Rims

Rims (Fig. 14.1):

- *Aortic—Superoanterior:* Best seen in aortic short axis view on 2D transthoracic view. Absent aortic rim usually did not stop device

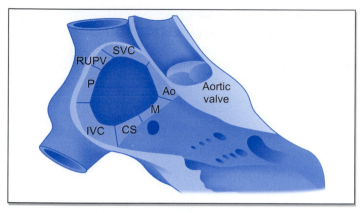

Fig. 14.1: Schematic representation of locations of rims in ASD

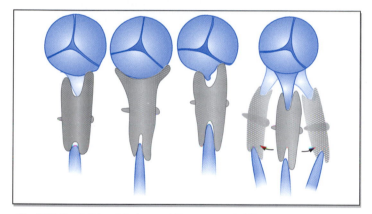

Fig. 14.2: Possibilities of device-straddling aorta with different aortic rim margins

closure, if other rims were present. The figure down and recent reports of aortic wall erosion has brought the necessity of this rim into consideration too (Fig. 14.2).

- Atrioventricular—mitral or inferoanterior
  The rim is best seen in A4C view in TTE and in TEE at 0°.
- Superior vena caval (SVC)—Superoposterior
  SVC and IVC rim—Best assessed in TEE at 45°. You might have to manipulate probe as mentioned in TEE section to look for IVC rim.
- Inferior vena caval (IVC)—Inferoposterior.
- Posterior—Posterior free wall of atria.
  A margin > 5 mm is considered adequate. Many morphological variations exists, the most common being deficient aortic rim (around 42.1%).

Transesophageal echocardiography is performed in three different planes
- **Transverse (0°):** The posterior and mitral rims are best evaluated in this view (Figs 14.3A to C).
- **TEE at 45°:** This view helps in assessing the posterior and the aortic rims and often assesses maximum size of defect.
- **TEE at 90°:** This view evaluates SVC and IVC rims. The margins can be evaluated by rotating the probe at same level (Figs 14.4A to C).

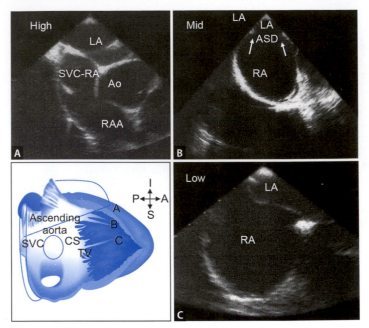

Figs 14.3A to C: At 0° we assess anterior and posterior rims as seen in Figure B. Here we demonstrate evaluating the defect completely by moving the probe in and out. In Figure (A) at the highest plane SVC—right atrial junction with intact septum is noted. The defect is well seen at mid level, while the septum reforms at lower level (C). This suggests that this septal defect is likely to have adequate margins for percutaneous closure

Steps of Closure

Few Tips

- Avoid taking up cases initially where transthoracic echocardiogram shows defect size > 35 mm
- *Role of balloon sizing:* Static balloon sizing of the ASD using NuMed PTS or AGA Amplatzer sizing balloon should be performed in the initial few cases, if there is slightest of doubt by noninvasive assessment. During balloon occlusion, color Doppler evaluation of the atrium septum to rule out additional atrial defects should be carried out.

Procedure

- Put a 7F sheath in femoral vein and a 5F sheath in femoral artery
- Perform routine right heart catheterization including saturation and pressure
- Cross the ASD with Cournand/Multipurpose/JRA catheter and 0.035" 'J' tipped Terumo guidewire. Park the wire in left upper pulmonary vein
- Exchange the guidewire for 0.035" Amplatz Superstiff 3 mm soft tip, 'J' tipped guide wire
- Exchange 7F sheath with 60–75 mm long compatible sheath
- Flush the sheath continuously when advancing
- Refrain from negative suction on these large sheaths

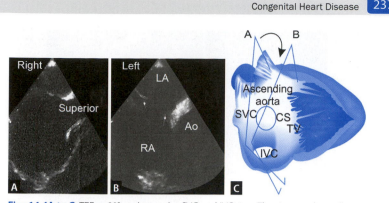

Figs 14.4A to C: TEE at 90° evaluates the SVC and IVC rims. The rims can be well seen by rotating the probe at same level. If the IVC rim cannot be seen, then the probe should be retroflexed after advancing into stomach. It should be withdrawn slowly between 70°–90°. As IVC-RA junction moves away, IVC will becomes perpendicular to ultrasound beam (Fig-III). We assess anterior and posterior rims as seen in Figure B. Here we demonstrate evaluating the defect completely by moving the probe in and out. In Figure (A) at the highest plane SVC—right atrial junction with intact septum is noted. The defect is well seen at mid level while the septum reforms at lower level. This suggests that this septal defect is likely to have adequate margins for percutaneous closure.

- Allow passive back bleed and keep the end of sheath significantly below the level of the patient's heart to facilitate bleed back
- Be aware of the patient's breathing and be sure to time clearance of sheath with exhalation to minimize risk of air embolism
- Give supplemental nasal cannula oxygen during sheath and device placement to minimize effects, if air embolism occurs
- Take the sheath till mid LA and remove wire and dilator and flush the sheath
- For large defects, tip should be positioned in the mouth of pulmonary vein
- Prepare the device by soaking it in heparinized saline. Inspect the device for any defects and constantly flush it while compressing it into loader/sheath to remove any residual air
- Position the tip of sheath in mid LA and release the distal disc of device
- Use TEE guidance to confirm the position. Make sure it is not opened in a pulmonary vein or pressed against LA roof.

Tips

Often the angle of sheath and atrial septum is very acute resulting in prolapse of LA disc. This mainly happens through anterosuperior region (aortic rim) or superior SVC region. To make device more perpendicular rotate the sheath clockwise to drive tip of sheath posterior and superior (Cook Inc has a sheath with posterior–superior curve called Lock-Hausdorf sheath). You can also use Amplatzer delivery sheath, which is supplied with the device.

Pull the device towards atrial septum and start releasing RA disk. The larger the defect the further the device center should be kept in LA during RA disk delivery to prevent LA disc prolapse into RA.

Perform complete echocardiographic assessment both in TEE and TTE (depending on comfort level) mode and angiographic views should

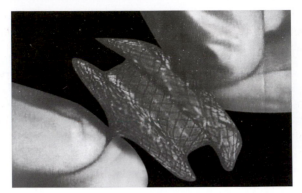

Fig. 14.5: Amplatzer septal occluder

be done. Look for any new onset TR/MR, residual left to right shunt and obstruction of SVC or pulmonary vein.

Perform slight pulling and pushing in delivery cable to separate the two discs and confirm stability. Release from delivery cable and remove the cable.

Observe the patient for 10 minutes. Maintain ACT > 250 seconds. and confirm that the patient is on Aspirin for 2 days prior to procedure.

Device Selection Tip

Oversize device by 3 or 4 mm from echo assessed size in defects more than 30 mm. For lesser defects, oversizing by 2 mm usually suffice. Total atrial chamber size and length of interatrial septum must be kept in mind while selecting device. Always use Amplatzer septal occluder in the initial cases (Fig. 14.5).

Ventricular Septal Defect Closure

Introduction

Ventricular septal defect (VSD) account for approximately 30% of all congenital heart disease. Because there is a high incidence of spontaneous closure of small VSDs, the incidence is much less in older infants and particularly in adults. There are four anatomic types of VSDs

1. Perimembranous or paramembranous (most common, about 80% of VSDs)
2. Muscular or trabecular (upto 15–20%)
3. Outlet supracristal or infundibular (approximately 5%)
4. Inlet or AVSD type (typically occurring in Down syndrome).

Indications for Percutaneous Closure of VSD (ACC/AHA, 2008 Guidelines)

- Qp/Qs > 2 or signs of left ventricular overload
- History of infective endocarditis
- Qp/Qs > 1.5 and when pulmonary artery pressure is less than two thirds of systemic pressure or the pulmonary vascular resistance is less than two-thirds of systemic vascular resistance, or there is left ventricular systolic or diastolic dysfunction.

Criteria for Percutaneous Closure

- Only type IV VSD or muscular defects are subjects to percutaneous closure, although there is extensive experience of type-II or perimembranous VSD.
- VSD following infarction for which surgery has been ruled out or in cases of postoperative residual shunt.
- Adequate rims (> 4 mm) from the defect towards the adjacent structures, including the aortic, pulmonary, mitral and tricuspid valves.

Contraindications for Percutaneous Closure

All septal defects, that are not muscular, such as type-I or sub-pulmonary defects, type-III defects or atrioventricular canal defects. There are doubts concerning type-II or perimembranous defects. Perimembranous defects with aortic valve prolapse or a markedly aneurysmal septum should be avoided. Other options should be considered in cases of nickel allergy, or contraindication for antiplatelet therapy.

Steps

1. Conscious sedation, heparin 100 units/kg (ACT 200–250 seconds), IV antibiotic.
2. Take access through right femoral artery and right femoral vein for perimembranous VSD. Take right internal jugular vein as access in addition to femoral artery in muscular VSD closure.
3. Left ventricular angiography in left anterior oblique/cranial projection to profile the VSD.
4. Cross the defect from left ventricular side by right Judkin's, multipurpose or Cournand catheter and 'J' tipped Terumo glidewire (exchange length).
5. Create an arteriovenous loop (AV loop) by snaring the wire in pulmonary artery and bringing it out from venous end.
6. Make sure the AV loop does not meet any resistance, is straight, without kinks on frontal image fluoroscopy. Otherwise repeat the step.
7. Advance long sheath (6–12 Fr) to the left ventricle from venous end. While using Torque delivery system, use 45° sheath (provided with Amplatzer device) for reaching middle of LV.
8. Deploy the occluder device under fluoroscopic and echocardiographic guidance (transesophageal echo preferable).

   A word about device
   Amplatzer muscular VSD occluder size ranges from (4–18 mm). Disc diameter is 8 mm more than waist (except 4 mm, where discs are 9 mm), length of waist is 7 mm. Select a device 2 mm larger than size assessed by TEE or angiography at end diastole (the biggest of 2 diameters).
9. Angiography in the left ventricle and ascending aorta to verify complete occlusion and appearance of any new aortic valve regurgitation.

Patent Ductus Arteriosus

Introduction

Patent ductus arteriosus (PDA) is the persistent communication between the proximal left pulmonary artery and descending aorta just distal to the left subclavian artery and accounts for 10% of congenital heart disease. In adults, it is usually an isolated finding. When a PDA occurs in isolation, device closure is usually feasible and can be successfully performed in the vast majority of adults with very low complication rate. Surgical closure of PDA in the adult is reserved for the patient with a duct too large for device closure or with inappropriate anatomy and where surgery is indicated for other concomitant cardiac lesions.

Indications for Intervention in PDA (ESC Guidelines, New Version, 2010)

Class I

1. PDA should be closed in patients with signs of LV volume overload.
2. PDA should be closed in patients with pulmonary arterial hypertension (PAH) but PAP < 2/3 of systemic pressure or PVR < 2/3 of SVR.
3. Device closure is the method of choice where technically suitable.

Class II A

1. PDA closure should be considered in patients with pulmonary arterial hypertension (PAH) and PAP > 2/3 of systemic pressure or PVR > 2/3 of SVR but still net left to right shunt (Qp:Qs > 1.5) or when testing (preferably with nitric oxide) or treatment demonstrates pulmonary vascular reactivity.
2. Device closure should be considered in small PDAs with continuous murmur (normal LV and PAP).

Steps of Device Closure

- The most common anatomical shape is conical with a large aortic ampulla that narrows at the pulmonary artery end, however, other distinct anatomical forms exist
- Different tools and techniques exist, but here we will focus on the two most common techniques for conical-shaped ductus
- For PDAs less than 3 mm retrograde placement of embolization coils, and for larger ducts, antegrade placement of Amplatzer duct occlusion is preferred
- Procedural success is resulting in complete closure is > 96% with complications occurring in less than 5%. Device embolization, thrombus and ductal aneurysm has been reported in < 1%
- After due consent, antibiotic prophylaxis take both femoral artery and venous access. 5 Fr. femoral artery is usually sufficient
- Perform angiogram of proximal descending thoracic aorta by pigtail catheter in straight lateral plane and RAO caudal (30/15°) view

- This will separate PDA from the descending aorta showing the distal transverse arch
- Cross the PDA from the MPA using JR4 catheter and floppy directional wire like 0.035" Terumo glidewire into proximal abdominal aorta
- Take an end-hole catheter over this guidewire, and exchange it for 0.035" 'J' tipped exchange wire (Amplatzer Superstiff)
- 6 or 7-Fr long sheath with a curved tip should be placed across the PDA into midthoracic DAO. Rotate the sheath clockwise as it moves into RVOT to avoid getting caught on the moderator band
- *Device selection:* Amplatzer duct Occluder device is a Nitinol wire mesh self-expanding device with a wider aortic flange measuring 2 mm larger than central duct plug that ranges in length from 5–8 mm. Central duct plug diameter ranges from 4–14 mm
- The diameter of ductal portion of the device should be 2 mm larger than the minimal diameter of the PDA. So a 3.7 mm minimal diameter ductus can be closed with 8–6 mm device
- Load the device and take it till the tip of sheath
- Pull the entire system till the tip of sheath is just off the posterior wall of the DAO at the level of ductal ampulla
- Holding the device in plane the sheath is retracted to open the distal flange only. Bony structures and tracheal air column should also be used as landmarks for delivery
- Withdraw the entire system such that the aortic flange is pulled firmly against the aortic ampulla
- Perform a lateral angiogram in thoracic DAO to confirm appropriate position of aortic end of device
- Retract the sheath holding the device cable in position to open the ductal plug within the PDA
- A hand angiogram through the delivery sheath to assess PA side of the device. If PA end protrudes > 3 mm or there is evidence of LPA obstruction, recapture the device
- Repeat pigtail angiogram in DAO to confirm appropriate device position. Unscrew the device keeping slight tension on the cable to maintain position
- A final angiogram through the pigtail catheter in the proximal thoracic DAO is performed in lateral projection (35 cc at 35 cc/sec) to assess final position and closure. Some leak through the device is expected as fibrin deposition on the fabric for complete closure occurs over hours
- Long- and bizarre-shaped PDAs may be occluded by coils—Amplatzer duct occluder or Amplatzer vascular plugs
- For simplicity sake Krichenko classification and other devices are not being discussed
- For PDAs less than 3 mm coil closure is preferred. Coil length should allow at least four loops (one loop on PA side and remainder in aortic ampulla). So length ≥ 4 × pie × loop diameter. For example, a 2.5 mm minimum diameter PDA can be closed by 0.038", 7 cm long, 5 mm loop diameter coil which will provide a total 4.4 loops. Loop diameter ≥ 2 times the minimal PDA diameter

- Place the JR4 retrogradely from femoral artery in the main PA. Place the roadmap image from lateral angiogram on left. A straight 0.035" wire used to load or the embolization coil into the catheter and advance or push the coil to the tip. Release the coil to take one loop on PA side, and then withdraw catheter over the pushing wire to uncover the proximal end of coil
- Perform angiogram after 10–15 min by hand keeping direction catheter at the tip of the inferior margin of the aortic ductal ampulla. If contrast passes through the coil as a jet and fills into the MPA, 5 mm or more part of the PA end, more coils will be required.

Complications of Percutaneous Coronary Intervention

■ Prithwiraj Bhattacharjee, Shuvanan Ray

Introduction

Percutaneous coronary intervention (PCI) has revolutionized the treatment of patients with coronary artery disease. It has the ability to relieve symptoms of angina in stable coronary disease and can modify the natural history of acute coronary syndromes (ACS). Being invasive in nature, it is a potentially hazardous procedure, especially if performed by the less experienced interventionist. Complications of this procedure are well described and may lead to fatal outcomes. A thorough knowledge about these complications and their management is a must before embarking on the procedure.

Types of Complications

Complications during PCI may occur at various stages. Here, we broadly classify them as:
- Complications related to vascular access,
- Coronary complications,
- Post-procedural complications, and
- Others.

Complications Related to Vascular Access

The common femoral artery (CFA) is the most frequently used vascular access for PCI. Compared to radial artery, CFA access has several advantages like larger vessel diameter allowing easier cannulation and introduction of larger guide catheters, thus helping in performing complex procedures. Although a relatively simple and safe procedure occurs in an experienced hand, complications do occur and range from small self-limiting hematomas to life-threatening retroperitoneal hemorrhage. Risk factors related to increased bleeding complications due to CFA access, are:
- Female gender
- Older age
- Obesity
- Low body weight
- Peripheral vascular disease
- Use of fibrinolytics
- Larger heparin dose
- Use of GP IIb/IIIa inhibitors
- Prolonged indwelling sheath time
- Larger sheath diameter.

Complications of Femoral Access

- Hematoma
- Pseudoaneurysm
- Retroperitoneal hemorrhage
- Femoral artery thrombosis
- Arteriovenous fistula
- Dissection
- Lower limb ischemia
- Neuropraxia.

Management of Complications

Hematoma

- *Femoral:* It is a collection of blood within soft tissues of upper thigh. Groin hematomas are the most common complications of femoral arterial puncture.
- *Clinically:* It is a tender mass of varying sizes at the femoral puncture site.
- Needs to be differentiated from pseudoaneurysm.
- Needs to be certain about continuous leak (increasing hematoma size).
- Ice-compression is helpful.
- May need blood transfusion.

Pseudoaneurysm

- Pulsatile mass over groin area with occasionally audible bruit as a result of blood accumulation around an unsealed arterial puncture.
- *Ultrasound necessary for confirmation of diagnosis:* Echolucent extraluminal cavity in communication with CFA with to and fro blood flow during systole and diastole.
- Pseudoaneurysms <2 cm may be treated conservatively as most of them resolve spontaneously.
- Larger symptomatic pseudoaneurysms need to be treated by surgical or nonsurgical procedures.
- *Nonsurgical management includes:*
  - Manual compression of the neck of aneurysm by ultrasound probe for 30–60 minutes (particularly for narrow neck)
  - Ultrasound-guided thrombin injection.
- *Indications of surgical repair of pseudoaneurysms:*
  - Infected pseudoaneurysms
  - Rapid expansion
  - Failure of other therapies
  - Skin necrosis
  - Compression syndromes
    - » Neuropathy
    - » Claudication
    - » Critical limb ischemia.

Retroperitoneal Bleed

- Unusual but potentially fatal
- Risk increases with high (above inguinal ligament) femoral puncture

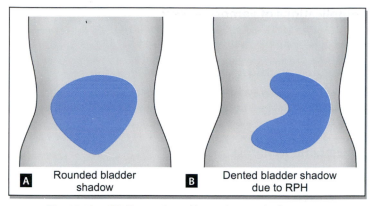

Figs 15.1A and B: Retroperitoneal hemorrhage under fluoroscopy

- Signs and symptoms of retroperitoneal bleeding usually consist of hypotension, nausea, vomiting, abdominal distension, fullness or abdominal pain.
- Diagnosis confirmed by abdominal/pelvic ultrasound or CT, a simple fluoroscopy in cathlab of the contrast-lined bladder can be used to diagnose retroperitoneal hemorrhage, which causes distortion of the shadow (Figs 15.1A and B).
- Stop anticoagulation and resuscitate with crystalloid/blood transfusion, vasopressor therapy.
- If no improvement, prolonged balloon inflation in the site of leakage or placement of a covered stent if the anatomy is suitable.
- Surgical repair when above methods fail/not applicable.
- Independent predictors of mortality in patients with retroperitoneal hemorrhage (Trimarchi, JACC, 2010).
  - Female sex
  - History of myocardial infarction
  - Cardiogenic shock
  - Pre-procedure creatinine ≥1.5 mg/dL
  - LVEF ≤50%.

Femoral Artery Thrombosis

- Can occur when a large sheath or catheter (e.g. IABP) has been placed in a small caliber femoral artery and kept for prolonged period.
- Pain, pallor, pulselessness in distal limb with impaired motor/sensory function—if not corrected promptly by sheath/catheter removal, should alert the operator.
- Limb flow must be restored within 2–6 hours to prevent muscle necrosis.
- Urgent vascular surgery consultation to explore and treat dissection or Fogarty catheter embolectomy of distal artery is necessary.
- Contralateral femoral access to address common femoral occlusion percutaneously.

Arteriovenous Fistula

- Risk increases with low femoral puncture below CFA bifurcation or with left-sided femoral puncture by right-handed operator.

- Usually asymptomatic.
- One third cases close spontaneously within a year.
- Initial conservative approach is advisable.

Neuralgic Complications

- May be extremely symptomatic, but usually benign.
- Usually caused by neuropraxia rather than nerve transection.
- Usually heals spontaneously by 6 months.

Lower Limb Ischemia

- Acute limb ischemia due to thrombosis/embolism is a limb threatening complication.
- Pulseless, pale, painful and paresthetic limb is an emergency.
- Diagnostic peripheral angiogram should be performed to locate the site of block.
- Catheter-guided locally administered thrombolytic agents such as tenecteplase, tPA, rt-PA or reteplase can be used as low-dose continuous infusion.

Protocol of Catheter-derived Thrombolysis

- Heparin 30 µ/kg at the onset of catheterization, then 3 µ/kg/hour through the arterial sheath
    - Tenecteplase   0.2 mg/hour
    - tPA   0.5 mg/hour   × 20 hours
    - rt-PA   0.2 µ/hour
- Surgical therapy includes balloon catheter thrombectomy (Fogarty catheter), open surgical thrombectomy or bypass.

Radial Access Complications

- Reduced hemorrhagic complications but requires a significant learning curve.
- Complications are:
    - Vasospasm
    - Pseudoaneurysms
    - Dissection/perforation
    - Compartment syndrome
    - Radial artery occlusion
    - Catheter kinking.

Management

- **Severe vasospasm:** Radial artery is muscular and rich in alpha-1 and alpha-2 adrenoceptors. Repeated local or distant stimulation or even patient's anxiety may induce spasm in radial artery. Prevention by a cocktail of intra-arterial nitrate and calcium channel blocker is an easier option than treatment of spasm. Sedation, analgesia, nitrate and calcium channel blocker in additional doses may be required to relieve severe spasm. Rarely regional anesthesia or deep sedation or general anesthesia by anesthetist may be required to remove the equipments without avulsion of artery.
- **Compartment syndrome:** Caused by raised pressure in a closed osseofascial space. Pressure >30 mm Hg gives rise to ischemia of

forearm muscle. Cardinal sign is pain during dorsiflexion. Early detection is important and proximal compression may limit hematoma and mitigate the situation. Any sign of neurovascular deficit warrants urgent fasciotomy and/or vascular surgery.

- **Pseudoaneurysm:** May occur rarely due to suboptimal post-procedure radial artery compression. Management is similar to femoral artery pseudoaneurysm.
- **Radial artery occlusion:** The risk of radial occlusion is high when there is inadequate anticoagulation, small diameter vessel, long duration post-procedural compression. However, there is no report of hand ischaemia following diagnostic or interventional transradial coronary procedure.
- **Catheter kinking:** Although catheter kinking may occur in femoral access, it is more common in radial access due to increased catheter friction and presence of loops. Catheter must not be withdrawn before straightening the loop by rotating it in the opposite direction and inserting a hydrophilic wire to bring the catheter in a larger artery.

How to reduce transradial access complications?
- Hydration and anxiolysis
- Vessel cocktail (calcium-channel blockers and nitrate)
- Heparin (at least 3000–5000 IU)
- Perfusion hemostasis
- Proper sheath size
- Avoid multiple exchanges of guide catheters.

Coronary Complications

Complications during the procedure may be related directly to the damage of coronary arteries or secondarily due to the hardwares used in the procedure. Direct injury to the coronary arteries may result in coronary perforation, coronary dissection or acute vessel closure/ no reflow phenomenon. Hardware-related complications include embolization of stent, balloon or broken guidewires.

Coronary Perforation

Perforation is an anatomical breach in the integrity of the tunica adventitia of an epicardial artery leading to extravasation of blood, either into the myocardium, pericardium or a cardiac chamber. In the majority of cases, perforation occurs as a complication of coronary angioplasty and is related to several possible mechanisms:

- Perforation of the arterial wall by guidewire (stiff wires, hydrophilic wires)
- During rotational atherectomy
- Excessive stretching of vessel wall by oversized balloon or stent.

The classification of coronary perforation proposed by Ellis et al. is widely accepted. It is an angiographic classification and described as the following types:

- *Type 1:* Extraluminal crater without extravasation. This type of perforations are generally without consequences and may be managed conservatively.
- *Type 2:* Pericardial or myocardial blush without contrast jet extravasation.
- *Type 3:* Extravasation through frank (>1 mm) perforation generally accompanied by tamponade and poor short-term prognosis.

- *Type 4 (Cavity spilling):* Perforation into an anatomic cavity/chamber. Usually, has a better prognosis compared to Type 3 frank perforation into pericardium.

  Predictive factors:
  - Old age
  - Female sex
  - Tortuous/calcified vessel
  - Small diameter vessel
  - Chronic total occlusion angioplasty
  - Saphenous vein graft angioplasty
  - Use of atherectomy device
  - Intravascular ultrasound use
  - Oversizing of balloon/stent (very important).

Management

Treatment of coronary perforation depends on the size of perforation, the extent of contrast medium extravasation and the hemodynamic status of the patient. Initial management should focus on the sealing of the perforation to prevent cardiac tamponade. This can be achieved by means of either prolonged balloon inflation or by a covered stent. Emergency echocardiogram should be done. Different strategies are discussed as follows:

- **Prolonged balloon inflation:** A balloon should be placed at the perforation site and inflated at minimum pressure to achieve hemostasis (usually <5 atm) for at least 10 minutes. Evaluation by repeated contrast injections, at intervals, is recommended. In case of incomplete sealing, use of a perfusion balloon catheter may allow prolonged inflation of 15–45 minutes with less ischemia.

  Reversal of heparin is not advised as long as the balloon and the wire is inside the coronary artery. Reversal of heparin with these devices inside the artery may cause thrombosis of the artery and severe ischemia. When the devices are withdrawn from the vessel, the reversal of heparin may be performed. GPIIb/IIIa receptor blockers, if running IV should be stopped in the beginning. Bivalirudin should be discontinued as it takes 2 hours for the coagulation parameters to come to normal.

- **Pericardiocentesis and reversal of anticoagulation:** Type 1 and 2 perforations are usually managed by balloon occlusion or by conservative approach. However, type 3 perforations require more aggressive management like pericardiocentesis.

- **Covered stent:** Polytetrafluoroethylene (PTFE) covered stents have been successfully used to treat coronary perforation when conservative approach fails. However, the profile of the stent is unsuitable for tortuous vessel anatomy or distal vessel.

  Placing a covered stent (Figs 15.2A to C):
  - Try from contralateral access.
  - Put another 7F guide (can take 6F guide if the stent is 6F compatible).
  - Try another guidewire to the proximal end of inflated balloon, now the balloon is deflated for brief period and cross the lesion with the wire and balloon inflated again.
  - Take the stent like the second wire and place across the lesion, remove the first wire and balloon and deploy the stent.

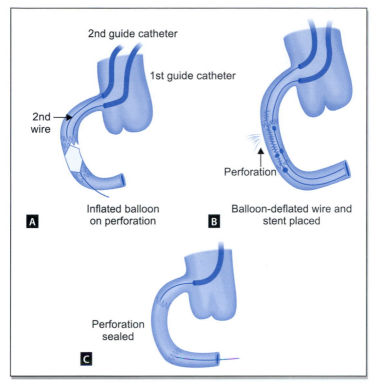

Figs 15.2A to C: Placing a covered stent

A few words about covered stents:

A turning point in the treatment of coronary perforations occurred with the introduction of covered stents (stent grafts), which allow for the percutaneous sealing of the rupture (Fig. 15.3) (Briguori et al. 2000; Lansky et al. 2006).

- **JOSTENT GraftMaster® (Abbott Vascular, Abbott Park, Illinois):** Stainless steel stent covered with polytetrafluoroethylene (PTFE); characterized by a wall thickness of 0.3 mm; available in sizes 3.0, 3.5, and 4.0 (6-Fr guiding catheter) and 4.5 and 5.0 (7-Fr guiding catheter). It is bulkier than the other covered stents.
- *In situ* **Direct-Stent® Stent-Graft (In situ Technologies Inc. St Paul, MN):** Stainless steel PTFE-covered stent; wall thickness 0.15 mm; it is the thinnest covered stents available (starting at 1.2 mm crossing profile; available in sizes from 2.5 mm diameter to 6.0 mm; minimum guiding catheter size ¼ 6–7 Fr).
- **Over and Under® Pericardium Covered Stent (ITGI Medical, or Akiva, Israel):** Stainless steel stent covered with equine pericardium (105 mm thickness); highly flexible stent available in sizes 2.5, 3.0, 3.5 (6-Fr guiding catheter); 4.0 mm (7-Fr guiding catheter). Theoretically, the equine pericardium may be more biocompatible reducing the risk of stent thrombosis.
- **PK Papyrus® covered Coronary Stent System (BIOTRONIK Inc., Berlin, Germany):** Cobalt Chromium stent platform single covered stent design with non-woven, electrospun polyurethane (90 μ thick); highly flexible stent available in sizes 2.5, 3.0,3.5,4.0

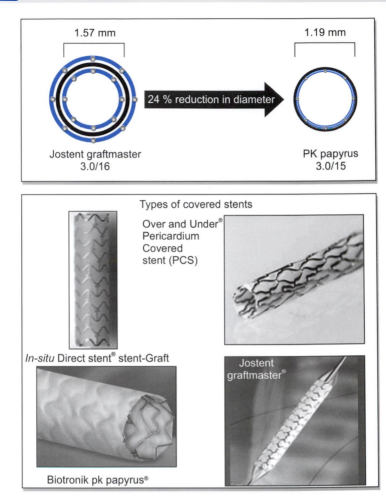

Fig. 15.3: Different covered stents

(5 Fguiding catheter); 4.5, 5.0 (6 F guiding catheter). Strut thickness of the stent varies from 60 µ (2.5, 3.0) to 120 µ (4.5, 5.0). Compared to Graftmaster®, it is less bulky and has smaller crossing profile.

Deploying a covered stent: A major drawback in treating a perforated vessel with a coronary stent graft is the amount of time that passes between the deflation of the sealing balloon and the final delivery of the covered stent into the lesion site. For this reason, we would always recommend the dual-guiding catheter technique for implantation of the covered stent (Ben-Gal et al. 2010). While the sealing balloon is inflated, the guide catheter is withdrawn slightly from the coronary ostia, and another 7-French guiding catheter from the contralateral femoral artery is used to engage the same coronary ostia. A coronary-covered stent graft (or a coil in smaller and distal vessels) is advanced on a new wire through the second guide and placed just proximally to the sealing balloon. The sealing balloon is deflated and withdrawn proximally to allow passage of the wire and of the coronary stent graft which is deployed.

Managing distal wire perforations:

- Distal wire perforations, compared to vessel rupture, are subtler, since the operator may not notice them immediately.
- Most often occur with the use of hydrophilic wires that have been advanced too distally.
- Operator should leave hydrophilic wires with a loop distally and that he/she should always monitor the guidewire position in the distal coronary artery with fluoroscopy when using hydrophilic, tapered, or stiff wires.
- If distal perforation occurs, the operator can perform distal balloon inflation, coil embolization, or microparticle injection (Godino et al. 2009).
- When distal wire perforation appears to resolve with only prolonged balloon inflation, the patient should be closely monitored for at least 48 h, since late bleeding and tamponade may, sometimes, occur.
- When microcoil embolization is used for distal perforations, the coils should be released as distally as possible, and the deployment should start within the pericardial space before retreating into the vessel in order to ensure successful hemostasis.
- For microparticle embolization, begin with 300–400 mm particles and to increase to 600–700 mm if effective embolization is not obtained (Stankovic and Colombo 2007; Godino et al. 2009).
- *Surgery:* When nonoperative measures fail to control ischemia and provide hemodynamic stability in large perforations, surgical ligation of the artery with bypass grafting may be required. An algorithm is provided below (Flow chart 15.1).

Flow chart 15.1: Algorithm of coronary perforation

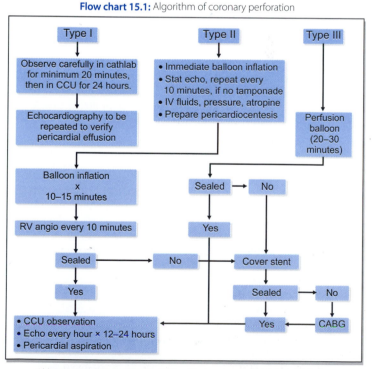

Abbreviations: IV, intravenous; CCU, critical care unit; RV, right ventricular; CABG, coronary artery bypass grafting

Coronary Dissection

Plaque fracture, intimal splitting and localized medial dissection are normal mechanisms of angioplasty. However, when dissection involves part of vessel away from the target lesion, it becomes a life-threatening complication. Dissections may be caused during the guide catheter and guide wire manipulation, or during balloon and stent inflation. Deep injury of the media with intraplaque hematoma and tissue flap may occlude the coronary blood flow. Procedural dissections usually are limited distal to the point of endothelial injury, but may also extend retrogradely to involve the coronary ostium. Morphologically, dissections are classified into the following types:

- *Type A*: Minor radiolucency within lumen during angiogram without dye persistency
- *Type B*: Parallel track or double lumen separated by a radiolucent area without dye persistence
- *Type C*: Extraluminal cap with dye persistence
- *Type D*: Spiral luminal filling defect
- *Type E*: New persistent filling defect
- *Type F*: Non A-E types that lead to impaired flow or total occlusion.

Cause of Dissection

- Wire-induced dissection
- Dissection during balloon inflation
- Stent-edge dissection
- Guide catheter-induced dissection
  - Ostium of the artery
  - Retrograde aortic dissection.

Guidewire-induced dissection: Usually, found in chronic total occlusion intervention. Parallel wire technique, stingray could be used to wire and re-entry into the main branch.

Guide catheter-induced dissection: Aggressive guide catheter handling can produce guide catheter-induced dissection and severe hemodynamic compromise. Ostia of LMCA or RCA, LIMA and retrograde aortic dissections—all are possible consequences of guide catheter-induced dissection.

Risk Factors of Catheter-induced Coronary Artery Dissection

- *Left main disease:* 14 of the 20 left main dissections were due to contact of the catheter with the plaque
- Amplatz-shaped catheters
- Acute myocardial infarction catheterization
- *Other possible factors:*
  - Catheter manipulations
  - Vigorous contrast injection
  - Deep intubations of the catheter within the coronary artery
  - Variant anatomy of the coronary ostia
  - Vigorous deep inspiration

Types of guide catheter-induced dissection:
- Abrupt closure
- Localized to ostium
- Antegrade into branches

Flow chart 15.2A: Management of guide catheter dissection

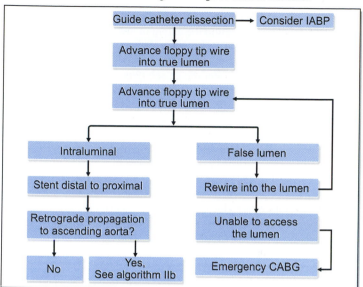

Abbreviations: IABP, intra-aortic balloon bump; CABG, coronary artery bypass grafting

Flow chart 15.2B: Dissection extending to aortic sinus

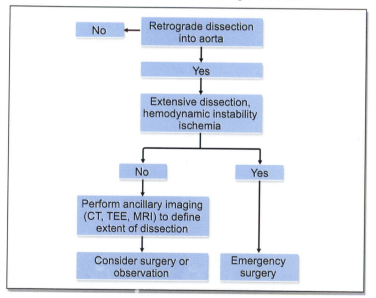

- *Retrograde (Dunning):*
    - Contrast staining only the coronary cusps
    - Contrast extends up the aortic wall up to 40 cm
    - Contrast extends up the aortic wall >40 cm

Management has been shown in Flow charts 15.2A and B.

Management

Outcome of coronary artery dissection and management depend on the patency of the distal vessel and the extent of propagation of dissection. In all cases, where there is extensive ischemia, IABP support should not be delayed.

1. *If there is abrupt closure of the vessel:* Urgent revascularization is mandated to prevent infarction of that myocardial territory. This may be achieved by coronary artery bypass grafting or PCI, the choice depends on the discretion of the operator.

2. *In absence of acute vessel closure:* If there is any suggestion of myocardial ischemia such as new ECG changes or chest pain, urgent revascularization should be undertaken to prevent myocardial infarction as that can occur even with TIMI II or TIMI III flow.

3. *Extent of propagation of dissection also alters management decision:* The dissections may be localized or they may extend in the antegrade or retrograde directions, resulting in scar formation and obstructing coronary flow. Extensive antegrade dissection can lead to acute vessel closure and most of the operators advocate that antegrade dissections be treated with PCI as soon as they are recognized.

Soft tip (floppy) wire with microcatheter should be used carefully to access the true lumen. Contrast should be injected through the micro-catheter to confirm location in the true lumen. If the initial attempt fails, the wire enters the false lumen, another floppy wire should be carefully manipulated into the true lumen.

- **Acute vessel closure/no-reflow phenomenon:** Abrupt vessel closure is one of the major complications of PCI. Most common cause of acute impairment of coronary perfusion is coronary dissection. Other causes are iatrogenic thrombus formation, embolization of native thrombus or atheroma, inadvertent injection of air or rarely coronary spasm.

  Iatrogenic thrombotic vessel occlusion: The causes are:
  - Multiple instrumentation with inadequate flushing of catheter
  - Suboptimal level of anticoagulation
  - Injection of thrombus formed in the guiding catheter
  - Use of reused hardwares.

    Management includes optimization of anticoagulation, intracoronary GPIIb/IIIa injection, mechanical thrombectomy. IABP insertion may be required to maintain hemodynamic stability.

Side Branch (SB) Occlusion

- Among the currently used technical approaches for bifurcation lesions is treatment with a single stent, that is, a planned stent implantation in the main vessel and stent implantation in the side branch, only if necessary. This simple approach is known as a provisional strategy.
- Occlusion of side branches has been reported in up to 20% of cases in which a stent was placed across a major (>1 mm) side branch (Aliabadi et al. 1997).
- In most cases, a greater than 50% stenosis was present at the ostium of the side branch, and most occlusions occurred after post-stent dilatation in the main branch with high-pressure inflations.

- In the COronary BIfurcation Stent II (COBIS II) study (stenting of 2,227 bifurcations of lesions with SB ≥2.3 mm), SB occlusion occurred 8.4%; independent predictors of SB occlusion are preprocedural percent diameter stenosis of the SB ≥50% and the proximal MV ≥50%, SB lesion length and acute coronary syndrome.
- In case of SB occlusion, flow was restored spontaneously in 13.9% and by SB intervention in 55.1%, but not 31.0%.
- Jailed wire in the SB is associated with significant higher rate of flow recovery (74.8% versus 57.8%) (Hahn et al. 2013).
- Bioresorbable vascular scaffold (BVS) is associated with a higher incidence of post-procedural SB occlusion compared with everolimus eluting metallic stent. This effect was more pronounced with small side branches with a reference vessel diameter ≤0.5 mm (Muramatsu et al. 2013).
- A study by Costa et al. (2012) has shown that side branch predilatation may be a feasible technique as it is associated with immediate side branch occlusion in <10% cases and the single predictor for failure was >85% stenosis of side branch at baseline.

Air Embolism

A complication common in the hand of junior interventionists in early months of training due to inadequate catheter aspiration, during manual injection via Y-connector or during equipment exchange. Rupture of PTCA balloon during angioplasty is another potential source. Helium from a ruptured IABP balloon is also a reported cause. More than half of these episodes are asymptomatic. However, even remarkably small amount of air (0.02 mL/kg) may cause unanticipated cardiac arrest. Symptoms such as chest pain with transient ST-elevation, arrhythmia culminating in VT or asystole may occur. Diagnosis is straightforward, when radiolucent bubbles traversing the coronary tree are seen in fluoroscopy or cineangiography.

Management

- Best treatment of inadvertent air injection is prevention.
- Meticulous checking of all connection of tubes for air bubbles before injection is the key of success.
- In a situation, where this unfortunate event takes place:
  - Administration of 100% O_2
  - Inotropic support to increase MAP/IABP
  - Suction of air bubble by thrombosuction catheter
  - Forceful injection of saline/patient's blood to propel air bubbles distally
  - Sometimes, prompt CPR may be life-saving.

Coronary Spasm

Coronary spasm during PCI in a reversible narrowing of the lumen of coronary arteries caused by tunica media smooth muscle hyperresponsiveness due to vasoconstrictor stimuli in a normal or diseased segment. It may occur following deep engagement of guide catheter, the passage of a stiff wire, balloon dilatation or stent deployment. It promptly responds to intracoronary nitroglycerin injection (200–800 µg). Intracoronary nicorandil is also an effective agent to treat vasospasm.

No-reflow Phenomenon

No-reflow phenomenon is defined as inadequate myocardial perfusion in the territory of a coronary artery without angiographic evidence of mechanical vessel obstruction. It typically accompanies primary PCI or complex angioplasty procedures like graft vessel angioplasty or use of rotational atherectomy device. Mechanism is likely multifactorial, like prolonged ischemia, reperfusion injury, distal embolization of thrombus or atheroma resulting in microvascular injury. Impaired TIMI (0-2) flow should raise the suspicion. Continued chest pain, lack of ST resolution in spite of TIMI 3 flow should alert the operator to assess myocardial blush. Predictors of no-reflow phenomenon during primary PCI are:

- High thrombus burden
- Lack of residual blood flow in IRA
- Prolonged ischemia
- Advanced age (>60 years), diabetes and hypercholesterolemia
- Reference vessel diameter >4 mm
- Lack of preinfarct angina (preconditioning).

Plan of Management: (See Chapter 12)

- Ensure no mechanical obstruction
  - Guide obstruction
  - Dissection
  - Distal macroembolus
  - Stent under-expansion
- IC vasodilators repeatedly
- Clear/Remove EPD, if it is in place
- Consider IC GPI (clear way?)
- Hemodynamic support
- Minimize additional mechanical intervention

Retained or Embolized Hardwares

The PCI equipment retained within circulation may include broken tip of guidecath, guidewire, balloon or stent.

- **Stent loss and embolization:** Even in the era of advanced stent design stent loss as a complication is not entirely eliminated. It usually occurs during pulling back of stentballoon assembly into the guidecath following unsuccessful attempt to cross the lesion, commonly due to heavy calcification, tortuosity or inadequate bed preparation.

Following strategies are employed (Figs 15.4A to F):

- **Deployment in the coronary circulation:** Possible when the guidewire is within the lost stent and stent can be deployed in a nonconsequential location by introducing a balloon within the uninflated stent.
- **Stent retrieval with balloon:** Most commonly attempted by passing a guidewire and small (1.5–2 mm) PTCA balloon distal to the stent and inflating the balloon distal to a stent at 1–2 atm pressure. The balloon is then gently pulled back along with the stent into the guiding catheter. Once the stent is secured in between the balloon

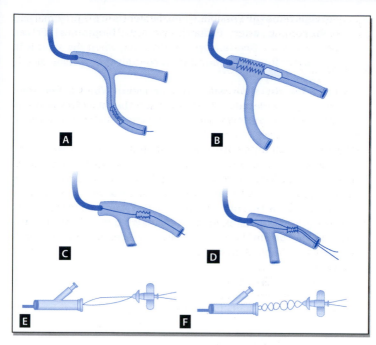

Figs 15.4A to F: Retrieval of lost stent with 'two wire technique': (A) If a stent is lost distally with a wire still across can probably best be left *in situ*, and gradually expanded from low profile to normal ballooning; (B) If a stent is lost proximally with wire across, the stent is crossed with small ballooning, then inflating distally and pulling the whole unit (wire + balloon + guide cath). Now two wires are put into a single torquing device: (C) Dislodged stent on wire; (D) A second wire is advanced through the stent strut; (E) Wires are torqued together forcing a helix; (F) Helix propagates distally and can be used to ensure a trapped wire fragment and then withdraw the whole unit

and guide catheter, the stent may be pulled back to iliac artery and removed through the arterial sheath. This technique is successful when there is no damage to the stent. Any resistance during pull back should prompt the operator to abandon the procedure.

– **Stent retrieval with snare:** Amplatz gooseneck snare with a right-angle snare loop is the preferable option. The position of the wire within the embolized stent helps in the retrieval technique. The snare is taken down over the angioplasty wire to the distal end of the stent, sometimes, with the help of a second wire, followed by advancement of transport catheter to tighten the loop around the stent. It can be withdrawn to iliac artery with the snare. The 6/7 F sheath may be exchanged for a 9F sheath at this point to facilitate the removal of the stent.

– **Free stent (not on wire) retrieval:** Proper alignment of the snare loop with the free end of the stent is necessary for successful retrieval. The plane of snare must be at right angle with the free end of embolized stent. The embolized stent should be seen in full length under fluoroscopy. Then the snare is held in such a way that only a straight line or the full closed loop of the snare is visible, confirming the vertical plane of alignment. This position allows capture of embolized stent. The next important step is to advance the transport catheter instead of pulling the ends of the snare which will cause disengagement of the stent.

- **Forceps removal:** Possible, when the stent is in the proximal part of the coronary artery. Pediatric myocardial bioptomes (3Fr) can be used. Not a first-line option. However, when the stent is in iliac artery forceps, removal from contralateral/ipsilateral side may be attempted.
- **Crushing the stent with another stent:** When a free stent cannot be retrieved, another stent may be taken to the site of embolization and deployed there, crushing the embolized stent against the wall.

- **Wire entrapment or fracture:** Entrapment can occur during bifurcation lesion procedures when two guidewires (main branch and side branch) are used, or during the use of a "buddy wire" to deliver a stent in a tortuous vessel. During stent deployment in the main branch, the side branch wire is "jailed" between the stent and the artery wall. High pressure post-dilatation before removal of the "jailed wire" or the "buddy wire" leads to wire entrapment. Once the wire is entrapped management depends on whether it is intact or fractured.
  - **Intact wire:** A small balloon loaded on the entrapped wire may be inflated at the proximal part behind the stent to release the wire. After removing the jailed wire a wire is placed distally through the stent and the stent is re-expanded by post-dilatations.
  - **Fractured wire:**
    » Small fractured segment totally behind the stent is kept as such. If a small segment is left uncovered, another stent is deployed over it.
    » If fractured entrapped segment extends into the guide catheter, then a balloon can be inflated within the guide cath or a stent can be deployed at high pressure within the guide cath, to hold the end of fractured wire and the whole system is then removed en block.
    » Long fractured segments removal by snaring is a technically challenging procedure and most of the time unsuccessful. Open surgical removal may be considered.
    » In presence of continued dual anti-platelet therapy, there is an argument to leave small fractured segments *in situ*.

- **Equipment knot:** Guide catheter knotting is more common during radial than femoral approach due to increased tortuosity in the peripheral vessel. Excessive torque movement delivered to the catheter shaft is the cause. Lack of movement in the catheter tip despite torquing along with pressure damping should alert the operator about this complication. By applying torque to the opposite direction under fluoroscopy, the knot can be removed. Passing a wire through the catheter, if possible, helps. If unsuccessful, a second access point (femoral for radial or vice versa) is established and the distal end of the catheter is snared. Application of opposite torque by the snare along with traction from both ends disentangles the knot. As a preventive measure, whenever there is extreme tortuosity, engagement of coronary ostia should be performed with guidewire within the guide catheter to stiffen the shaft of catheter. Use of long sheath is another precautionary measure.

Post-procedural Complications

Contrast-induced Nephropathy (CIN)

Contrast-induced nephropathy is defined as either 25% increase of serum creatinine from baseline or absolute increase of 0.5 mg/dL or higher in serum creatinine level with a reduction of urine output to < 0.5 mL/kg/hour for 6 hours after percutaneous cononary intervention using a contrast agent. The most important risk factors for CIN are impaired renal function (CrCl <60%), diabetes and reduced intravascular volume. CIN leading to dialysis has a very poor in hospital and 2-year survival (36% and 81% mortality respectively) (Flow chart 15.3).

- **Pathophysiology:**
  - Direct toxicity of iodinated contrast material to nephron
  - Microshower of atherothromboli to kidney
  - Contrast material and atheroemboli-induced renal vasoconstriction
    A clinical prediction rule is available to estimate the risk of nephropathy.

Flow chart 15.3: A sample algorithm for risk stratification, potential prevention, and assessment of CI-AKI occurrence

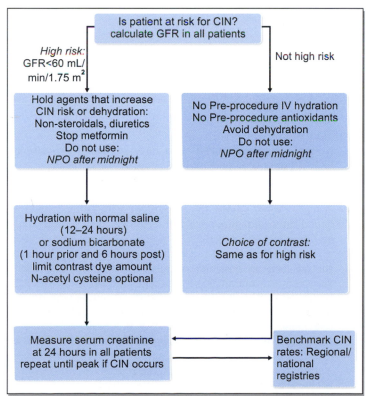

Abbreviations: CIN, contrast-induced nephropathy; NPO, nothing by mouth; GFR, glomerular filtration rate (*https://doi.org/10.1161/CIRCULATIONAHA.110.953851*)

- **Risk Factors:**
  - Systolic blood pressure <80 mm Hg—5 points
  - Intra-arterial balloon pump—5 points
  - Congestive heart failure (Class III-IV or history of pulmonary edema)—5 points
  - Age >75 years—4 points
  - Hematocrit level <39% for men and <35% for women—3 points
  - Diabetes—3 points
  - Contrast media volume—1 point for each 100 mL
  - Renal insufficiency:

  Serum creatinine level >1.5 g/dL—4 points

  or

  Estimated glomerular filtration rate (online calculator)
  - 2 for 40–60 mL/min/1.73 m^2
  - 4 for 20–40 mL/min/1.73 m^2
  - 6 for < 20 mL/min/1.73 m^2
- **Scoring:**
  - 5 or less points
  - Risk of CIN—7.5%
  - Risk of dialysis—0.04%

  - 6–10 points
  - Risk of CIN—14.0%
  - Risk of dialysis—0.12%

  - 11–16 points
  - Risk of CIN—26.1%
  - Risk of dialysis—1.09%

  - >16 points
  - Risk of CIN—57.3%
  - Risk of dialysis—12.8%
- **Prevention:**
  - A number of randomized trials have compared iso-osmolar, high-viscosity contrast with low-osmolar, low-viscosity contrast with varying results. Recently, the Cardiac Angiography in Renally Impaired Patients (CARE) trial randomized 414 patients at high risk for CI-AKI to angiography with either iopamidol or iodixanol; no difference in any measure of CI-AKI could be discerned between these 2 groups. Meta-analysis of these trials supports equivalent safety of iso-osmolar and low-osmolar contrast, with the possible exceptions of ioxaglate and iohexol.
  - Limit contrast volume (30 mL for diagnostic and 100 mL for PCI)
  - Hydration starting 3–12 hours prior to procedure with normal saline or isotonic sodium bicarbonate (at least 300–500 mL IV fluid before contrast injection).
  - Post-procedure hydration with target urine output of 150 mL/ hour
  - Avoid NSAIDs, metformin, aminoglycoside antibiotics
  - *N-acetylcysteine (NAC):* 600–1200 mg prior to PCI and 600 mg BD for 48 hours after PCI (role is controversial).

Stent Thrombosis

Most dreaded post-procedural complication of PCI is early stent thrombosis. Early stent thrombosis may be acute (<24 hours) or subacute

Table 15.1: Definitions of stent thrombosis

Definite stent thrombosis	Probable stent thrombosis	Possible stent thrombosis

Angiographic confirmation of stent thrombosis:
• The presence of a thrombus that originates in the stent or in the segment 5 mm proximal or distal to the stent, and at least 1 of the following within a 48 hour time window:
  – Acute onset of ischemic symptoms at rest
  – New ischemic ECG changes that suggest acute ischemia
  – Typical increase and decrease in cardiac biomarkers
Pathogenic confirmation of stent thrombosis:
• Evidence of recent thrombus within the stent determined at autopsy or via examination of tissue retrieved following thrombectomy
	• Any unexplained death within the first 30 days
	• Irrespective of the time after the index procedure, any MI that is related to documented acute ischemia in the territory of stent thrombosis and in the absence of any other obvious cause
		Any unexplained death from 30 d after intra-coronary stenting

(1–30 days). Although the incidence is lower (0.5–2%), the mortality is as high as 45%. Both the BMS and DES induce platelet adhesion, activation and thrombus formation. Effective antiplatelet therapy is mandatory after stent implantation until there is complete endothelialization of stents. Cytotoxic drugs in DES inhibit endothelialization and, therefore, risk of late (>30 days) and very late (> 1 year) stent thrombosis is higher with DES (Table 15.1).

Risk Factors:

Procedure- and lesion-related parameters:
- Use of multiple stents
- Small vessel diameter
- Coronary dissection
- Geographic miss
- Slow flow
- Long lesions
- Stent malapposition
- Under expansion of the stent.

Patient characteristics:
- Diabetes
- Acute coronary syndromes (especially STEMI)
- Left ventricular dysfunction
- Renal failure
- Advanced age
- High platelet reactivity.

Antiplatelet therapy:
- Inadequate intensity of therapy (i.e. non-dual platelet inhibition or insufficient dose)
- Noncompliance
- Premature cessation of antiplatelet therapy.

Management:
- Emergency thrombosuction
- Use of GPIIb/IIIa inhibitors
- Check platelet reactivity, if clopidogrel resistant, then shift to prasugrel/ticagrelor.

Coronary Aneurysm

- Coronary artery aneurysms after PCI are rare, with a reported incidence of 0.3–6.0%, and most 'aneurysms' are in fact pseudoaneurysms rather than true aneurysms.
- Coronary aneurysms have been reported from 3 days to up to 4 years after DES implantation procedures, with varying clinical presentations.
- Aneurysms after PCI are more commonly reported after ablative techniques particularly excisional atherectomy, residual dissection and deep arterial wall injury caused by oversized balloons or stents and high-pressure balloon inflations.
- DES stents inhibit neo-intimal growth by eluting the drug locally, delay re-endothelialization, and further may influence the remodeling process and lead to late incomplete stent apposition. Moreover, DES stents may aggravate inflammation and elicit hypersensitivity reactions leading to aneurysm formation.
- Inapparent bacteremia occurs frequently (in approximately 4–7% of cases) after complex percutaneous coronary intervention (PCI) with rare sequelae of infective aneurysm which is often fatal.
- Coronary intervention-associated aneurysms usually are detected at the time of repeat angiography for recurrent symptoms or as part of routine angiographic follow-up as mandated by study protocols. Coronary angiography is the gold standard for the diagnosis of coronary aneurysms, which are defined as a luminal dilatation 50% larger than that of the adjacent reference segment.
- Intravascular ultrasound (IVUS) has become the "gold standard" in providing critical diagnostic information to address these anatomic considerations in the evaluation of coronary aneurysms. Furthermore, other advanced coronary imaging techniques, such as computed tomography angiography, coronary magnetic resonance angiography, and real-time 3-dimensional echocardiography, also can be used as tools to detect and follow certain coronary aneurysms noninvasively.
- Treatment of coronary aneurysms be "individualized" using a combination of aneurysm size, expansion history, pathophysiology, and symptoms to decide when and if to apply therapy alternatives.
- Expanding pseudoaneurysms, infected aneurysms, and large, chronic (and expanding) aneurysms with symptoms should be treated.
- Concerns relating to stent graft treatment of coronary aneurysms include closure of contiguous side branches arising next to the aneurysm site, stent thrombosis, and recurrent restenosis.

- Placing coronary coils behind stents to thrombose the aneurysm sac can also be challenging and requires considerable expertise.
- Immediate surgical therapy for any confirmed infected aneurysm is recommended.

Stent Fracture (SF)

- There has been an increasing awareness of stent fracture (SF) as a potential complication following DES implantation.
- The majority of studies report the incidence of SF between 1 and 8%.
- Although most SFs occurred in sirolimus stents, several cases of SF were also reported in other types of stents, including BMS, Taxus and everolimus-eluting stent and zotarolimus (Table 15.2).

Predictors of Stent Fracture

- **Technical factors:**
  - Balloon or stent overexpansion, as it may theoretically weaken the stent struts.
  - Stent overlap, which results in localized rigidity creating hinge points that deform the stent leading to fracture.
  - *Stent length:* Longer stents may be subjected to higher radial forces.
  - Inappropriate handling of stent.

Table 15.2: Classification of SF according to different studies

Lee et al.	*Minor:* Single-strut fracture
Shaikh et al.	*Moderate:* Fracture >1 strut
Kim et al.	*Major:* Complete separation of stent segments
Umeda et al.	*Complete fracture:* Complete separation of stent segments
	Partial fracture: Single or multiple stent strut fracture
Chung et al.	*Disruption:* Inner and outer stent struts separated without displacement; linear or curvilinear alignment of stent maintained
	Avulsion: Outer struts separated; connection of inner struts maintained
	Displacement: Proximal and distal pats of fractured stents completely separated; linear or curvilinear of the stent lost
Lee et al.	*Avulsion:* Fractured sent segments separated completely (fluoroscopy) or stent struts absent from stent fracture site (IVUS)
	Partial: Stent struts absent in ≥1/3 of the vessel wall on IVUS
	Collapse: Folded and compacted inner and outer walls of the stent found in a bended segment with ≥ 45° on fluoroscopy
Nakazawa et al.	*Type 1:* Single-strut fracture
	Type 2: ≥2 strut fractures without deformation
	Type 3: ≥2 strut fractures with deformation
	Type 4: Multiple strut fracture with acquired transaction but without gap
	Type 5: Multiple strut fracture with acquired transection with gap in the stent body

Abbreviations: SF, stent fracture; IVUS, intravascular ultrasound.

– Stenting technique: An example of stenting technique that might cause SF is crush technique. A case has been reported of stent strut fracture in a bifurcation lesion treated with crush stenting, resulting in restenosis.

- **Stent type and stent conformability:** Stent conformability is defined as the degree to which a stent can bend around its longitudinal axis after deployment. Decreased stent conformability can lead to longitudinal straightening of the vessel after stent deployment, which subjects the stent to the countervailing force of the vessel wall. This tends to revert the vessel axis to its original shape, leading to SF.

- **Anatomic and pathologic factors which include the following:**
  – Tortuous and highly angulated vessel
  – Long lesions
  – Change in vessel angulation after stent implantation, which can create a significant distortion force
  – Complex lesions: In the ACROSS/TOSCA 4 study, SF was more frequent in the complex lesion subset of chronic total occlusion.
  – Stent location: SF is more common in right coronary artery (RCA) and saphenous graft locations as these vessels are dynamic during cardiac contractions. Stents in these locations may be subjected to repetitive distorting forces, as some segments of these vessels have more flexion points during the cardiac cycle. Repetitive cardiac contraction exposes the stent to compression, torsion, kinking, elongation, bending, and shear stress, which can cause fracture from mechanical fatigue. The points of SFs are usually located at hinges subjected to either medial or shear forces created by non-uniform vessel anatomy.

- **Other possible causes:** There are other possible causes that may lead to SF. Sanchez et al. reported a case of biventricular pacing leading to LAD coronary SF where the chief risk for SF was the vascular angulation; however, this risk was increased by abnormal myocardial contraction patterns that were induced by the ventricular pacing. Hoshi et al. reported a case of fatal ostial right coronary artery SF, aneurysm formation, and coronary artery perforation caused by mechanical stress between the sternum and dilated aortic root. SF was also reported following stenting of myocardial bridge. In one study, chronic kidney disease was found as an independent predictor of DES fracture.

Stent Fracture and Coronary Aneurysm

In an intravascular ultrasound (IVUS) study which was done to identify SF as a cause of stent failure, 17 patients were evaluated by IVUS, where 20 SFs were found. Five SFs occurred in a coronary aneurysm (accompanied by malapposition in three patients) despite the absence of aneurysm at index stenting. Comparing the SFs associated with aneurysm (5/20) with those that occurred without association with aneurysm (15/20), complete SF was more frequent (100% vs. 27%). All fractures were after Cypher-stent implantation and all presented more than 1 year after index stenting. It is possible that the association between coronary aneurysm and SF is a reciprocal one. In other words, as SF might cause aneurysm, aneurysmal formation and malapposition might precede SF. This would lead to excessive motion of the stent, leading to SF.

Diagnosis

- **Conventional fluoroscopy:** Stent visibility is limited on conventional fluoroscopy. There are several factors that contribute to stent visibility, including the patient's build, a stent platform, and stent thickness. Earlier generation stainless steel stents are more visible than the newer cobalt-chromium stents (such as Xience).
- **IVUS:** In several studies, IVUS was used to confirm the diagnosis of SF that was suggested by angiography. In other studies, IVUS detected several cases of SF that were missed by angiography. So, the use of IVUS increased the rate of SF detection in multiple studies. Another advantage of IVUS over conventional angiogram is the ability of IVUS to identify mechanisms of stent failure by providing information regarding neointima formation, vessel remodeling, perivascular tissue, stent expansion, stent strut distribution, and malapposition. A limitation of IVUS is that the resolution is not always good and the echoes frequently cause artifacts.
- **Stent boost:** This technology has improved the visibility of stent struts. It involves the automated detection of proximal and distal markers of balloon catheters in each cine frame. This automated marker detection is done through the identification of blob-like structures. This technology can also be used to position a stent precisely over a previously stented segment. Another advantage of stent boost over IVUS is that it does not add to the procedural costs. A limitation of stent boost technology is that a balloon catheter needs to be placed in the vicinity of a stent or stented segment in order to acquire images.
- **MDCT:** Compared to conventional catheter angiography, CTA has a higher accuracy for detection of SF.
- **OCT:** This imaging modality can also be used to detect SF. It was found that the absence of stent strut was the most common morphological feature of SF in OCT. The advantage of OCT over IVUS is that it has better resolution (10 times the resolution of IVUS) and fewer artifacts.

Management

There is no consensus about the ideal management of SFs. The decision should depend on the type of fracture, presence of ischemia, and the presence of factors that predict possible recurrence. If the reason of SF was stent overexpansion, then re-stenting the lesion again is possible with avoidance of stent overexpansion. On the other hand, when SF is caused by a non-modifiable factor like excessive vessel tortuosity, then referring the patient for CABG is more reasonable when there is a clear need for revascularization.

Others

Other important peri-procedural complications of PCI are:

Cerebrovascular Complications

- Main cause of catheterization-related stroke is embolic.
- Source of emboli is commonly atherosclerotic plaque at the aortic root, or may be emboli from LV thrombus.

- Inadequate anticoagulation, faulty catheter flushing or inadvertent air bubble introduction, placement of catheters or wires in arch vessels, are potential causes of stroke.
- For major hemispheric events, urgent carotid angiogram and neurovascular rescue should be considered.
- Patients receiving aggressive anticoagulation or thrombolytics are prone to spontaneous intracranial hemorrhage.
- Early recognition, prompt neurological consultation and CT scanning are necessary for better outcome.

Allergic and Anaphylactoid Reactions

- Precipitated by local anesthesia, iodinated contrast agent or protamine sulfate.
- Local anesthetics: Less common with lidocaine or bupivacaine, more common with procaine. Reactions to preservatives may also be the cause. Separate class of anesthetics or preservative-free anesthetics are to be used if there is history of allergy to a specific anesthetic.
- Iodinated contrast agents: Most common agent to trigger anaphylactoid reaction during PCI. Urticaria, angioedema of lips and eyelids, bronchospasms or shock. Premedication is recommended for patients with strong history of atopic reactions. A commonly practiced regime is steroid, antihistaminic agent and H_2 blocker before contrast injection. In case of severe reaction, 1 mL of 1:10,000 epinephrine diluted further to a total volume of 10 mL is injected IV in boluses of 1 mL every minute until arterial pressure is restored.
- Protamine sulfate: Common in IDDM patients receiving protamine insulin. Due to its restricted use in present-day practice, the incidence is very low.

Vasovagal Reactions

- One of more common complications (roughly 3% incidence) seen in cathlab.
- Triggered by pain and anxiety particularly in the setting of hypovolemia.
- Characterized by bradyarrhythmia associated with hypotension, nausea and sweating.
- Most of the incidences occur during securing of vascular access and removal of arterial sheath.
- Cessation of painful stimulus, rapid volume administration and atropine 0.6–1 mg IV is the treatment.
- It is important to remember that vagal stimulation is one of the earliest findings in perforation as the pericardium is irritated by the blood.

Arrhythmias

Ventricular Tachyarrhythmia

- Ventricular ectopy or even nonsustained VT is not uncommon during PCI.

- Passage of catheters into the ventricle or position of the guidewire in a small intramyocardial (septal) branch may initiate VT.
- Forceful injection of ionic (high-osmolar) contrast media in right coronary or its conus branch may initiate VT.
- Ischemia reperfusion-induced ventricular tachyarrhythmia is a common occurrence during PCI of ACS.
- Prolonged injection performed with partially damped catheter pressure can initiate VT.
- Unstable VT or VF must be treated by DC shock (200 joules increased to 300 joules, and if necessary to 360 joules).

Bradyarrhythmia

- Transient slow heart rate may occur commonly during PCI, especially during balloon inflation in inferoposterior infarction.
- RCA-related PCIs are often associated with sinus bradycardia or AV block, which is mostly reversible (vagally mediated involving SA node and proximal AV conduction system), whereas AV block associated with LAD territory infarct or PCI indicate large area of damage involving His-Purkinje system and often nonreversible.
- Sinus bradycardia usually does not require treatment unless it causes hemodynamic compromise.
- Atropine 1–2 mg IV usually adequate to treat bradycardia.
- In case of AV block, temporary pacing may be necessary.

Post-PCI thrombocytopenia (Flow chart 15.4)

- Thrombocytopenia following PCI is an underappreciated condition that is often clinically challenging. Its incidence ranges between 0.5% and 13% (Topol et al. 2001).
- Antithrombotic agents, such as unfractionated heparin (UFH), low-molecular-weight heparins (LMWHs), direct thrombin inhibitors, and antiplatelet therapies, such as thienopyridines, and platelet GPIIb/IIIa inhibitors, can all cause thrombocytopenia.
- Intra-aortic balloon pump (IABP) is an important therapy that is commonly associated with the development of thrombocytopenia in this setting.
- *Pseudothrombocytopenia* is an *ex vivo* artifact resulting from agglutination of platelets when the calcium content is decreased by blood collection in ethylenediaminetetraacetic acid (EDTA)-containing tubes. More than 30% of all cases of thrombocytopenia is attributable to pseudothrombocytopenia (Bizzaro 1995).
- *Heparin-induced thrombocytopenia (HIT):* A prothrombotic disorder initiated by heparin administration and is related to antibody-mediated platelet activation (IgG antibodies against platelet factor 4), causing thrombin generation and thrombotic complications.
- The "4Ts" of HIT refer to the degree of thrombocytopenia, the timing of the platelet fall after heparin exposure, the presence of thrombosis, and other causes for thrombocytopenia excluded (Strutt et al. 2011).
- Administration of GPIIb/IIIa antagonist (abciximab, eptifibatide, and tirofiban) is associated with an incidence approximately of 1–2%.

Flow chart 15.4: Laboratory testing to determine the cause of post-PCI thrombocytopenia

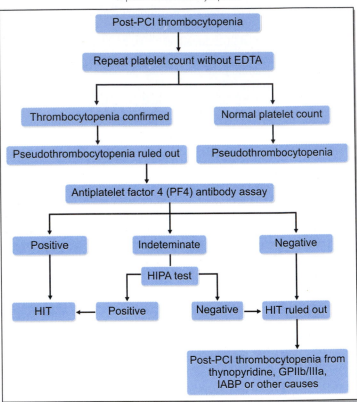

Abbreviations: EDTA, ethylenediaminetetra-acetic acid; GPI, glycoprotein IIb/IIIa inhibitor; HIPA, heparin-induced platelet activation; HIT heparin-induced thrombocytopenia; IABP, intra-aortic balloon pump; PCI, percutaneous coronary intervention

Source: Godino C, Colombo A. Complications of percutaneous coronary intervention. Pan Vascular Medicine. DOI 10.1007/978-3-642-37393-0_78-1)

- Eptifibatide and tirofiban have been associated with a lower occurrence of thrombocytopenia and bleeding compared to abciximab (Topol et al. 2001; Tcheng et al. 2000).
- Unfortunately, there are no guidelines on the management of patients with this condition.

Radiation Injury

- Patients undergoing PCI receive higher dose of radiation compared to diagnostic radiography.
- Prolonged fluoroscopy places the skin at high risk of injury like erythema, epilation, desquamation, ulceration and dermal necrosis.
- Risk is higher when fluoroscopic time is higher than 60 minutes and relatively fixed gantry position throughout the procedure.
- Controlling the fluoroscopic time is the direct responsibility of the operator.
- Total dose can be minimized through optimization of technical factors such as source to skin distance, angulation, minimum distance between the patient and image intensifier, etc.

Infections

- Although infections are not common during PCI, bacteremia has been reported after prolonged or complex PCI procedures.
- There have been isolated reports of life-threatening stent, groin or disseminated infection.
- Proper surgical scrubbing should be performed during procedure. Operator must wear surgical cap/mask.
- Routine antibiotic prophylaxis before PCI is not recommended.
- Risk of exposure of the operator to blood-borne infections like hepatitis B or HIV should be strongly considered and universal precaution must be taken to reduce risk of exposure.

Conclusion

One of the most important ethics of practicing medicine is primum *non nocere* (do no harm). A few rules, if followed stringently in practice, can save the young interventionist from a lot of troubles. These are the golden rules of PCI:

- Select your patient and the lesion carefully, plan in advance and anticipate problems.
- Have a thorough knowledge of your hardwares.
- Assess the angiogram and acquire adequate views before and after the procedure.
- Keep the procedure simple.
- Know your own limitation.
- Know where to stop.
- Do not stent a lesion just because 'it is there'.
- When something goes wrong, keep calm, pause for a moment, to think the best way out.
- Be focused all the time during the procedure.
- Learn from your own and other's mistakes and misfortunes.
  Best of luck!

Suggested Reading

1. Boyle AJ, Chan M. Catheter-induced coronary artery dissection. Journal of Invasive Cardiology. 2006;18(10).
2. Complications of cardiovascular procedures: Mauro Moscucci. Lippincott Williams & Wilkins, 2011.
3. Khan. Coronary air embolism. Catheter Cardiovascular Diag. 1995;36:313-8.
4. Meisel SR. A technique to retrieve stents dislodged in coronary artery. Cathet. Cardiovasc. Intervention. 2000;49:77-81.

Index

Page numbers followed by *f* refer to figure and *t* refer to table